Everything You Need to **Lose Body Fat, Shape Up,** *and* **Feel Great!**

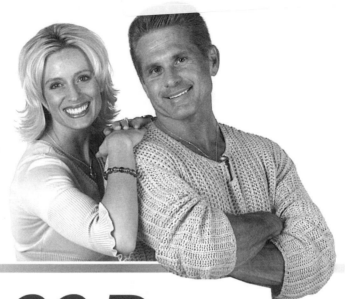

60 Day
PERSONAL POWER
HEALTH & FITNESS
Journal

John E. Peterson
& Wendie Pett

BRONZE BOW PUBLISHING

TABLE OF CONTENTS

INTRODUCTION

Dear Friend,

Wendie and I want to congratulate you on purchasing our *60 Day Personal Power Health and Fitness Journal.* The fact that you are reading this proves you have the seed of greatness inside you, and together we'll make it grow.

You are now entering what could easily become the most Transformative time of your entire life. During the next eight and one half weeks you will see and feel great changes occurring within your body and mind. If you are over-weight (and by that we mean over-fat), you will learn everything necessary to take complete control over your nutritional and exercise habits to give yourself the lithe, sculpted, slim look you have always desired.

You'll learn how to burn off body fat speedily while replacing much of it with beautifully shaped muscle. If you are underweight, you will soon start to add perfectly sculpted muscle mass to your body and feel a new sense of strength, power, and self-mastery. In short, you will start to create the body and life you've always dreamed of having instead of just dreaming about it.

Sounds great, doesn't it? Here's what we'll do to make it happen on the hurry up.

THE PERSONAL POWER HEALTH AND FITNESS JOURNAL

First of all, we provide a simple, brief course in healthy living. You will discover how to eat for radiant health and energy. Just that step alone can transform your health. Then we show you a foundational, basic fitness program that will develop dynamic strength and personal character through exercise. If you take charge of your eating habits and fitness, you'll be amazed at the masterful outlook it will give you on your entire life. You will be provided with everything you need to know to take yourself from where you are now to where you want to be.

This information is not, however, a substitute for the advice of a competent medical professional. If you have any questions or doubts about the advisability of following any advice herein, don't hesitate to consult your physician. And we advise you to always consult with your health practitioner before undertaking any new exercise or nutritional regimen. If there is any reason whatsoever that sensible exercise or change in diet could endanger your health, Don't Do It. Never. Consult your healthcare professional first, regardless of your age.

You may be wondering what the difference is between the information contained in this journal and the comprehensive Transformetrics™ Training System as taught by Wendie and me in our respective books, *Every Woman's Guide to Personal Power* and *Pushing Yourself to Power.*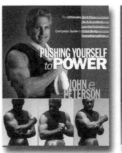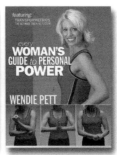
Basically, this journal is a guided course to healthy living and physique and figure enhancement, but not a substitute for the Transformetrics™ Training System. It will help you develop a physique to be proud of, most certainly. But it is only a small selection of some of the best that Transformetrics™ offers.

Once you have studied this information, you will know exactly what you need to do to achieve radiant health, strength, and lifelong vitality. You will *never* need to buy a single piece of exercise equipment, pay a single dime for a gym fee, or use drugs, chemicals, or gadgets of any kind, because your body will be your gym.

Not everyone desires or needs to achieve off-the-charts levels of strength and fitness. This journal contains a number of simple yet highly effective exercises that can and will benefit virtually everyone. This course will be your guide for the next 60 days. Where you decide to go then is entirely up to you!

Although continuing on in the Transformetrics™ Training System is a natural progression from this guided journal, it is in no way compulsory. We hope that you are so pleased with the results from this abbreviated version of Transformetrics™ that you decide to purchase our other books and DVDs in order to learn the entire system. If you do, we assure you that you will delighted with the benefits you receive from the full system of instruction. Regardless of what you decide, Wendie and I invite you to come to our web site and become a member of our Wendie Pett and John Peterson authors' forum. It is free of charge, and you'll learn a great deal about lifelong health, strength, and fitness from friends around the globe.

For now, though, let's focus on this course of instruction and your Transformation for the next 60 days. Although this course and journal may appear simplistic, if you *persist* in following these instructions to the letter, the results you desire *will* be achieved. It's a matter of natural law.

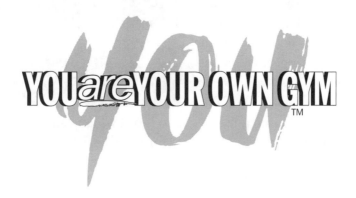

WHO CAN USE THIS COURSE AND JOURNAL

Whether you are young or not so young, male or female, thin or fat, muscular or weak, the methods of this course and journal *will* work for you. The great thing about Transformetrics™ is that it is continually self-adjusting to your current standard of fitness. As you become stronger and fitter, you will discover your musculature meeting its added demands *naturally*.

When we were born, our body was given to us as a gift from our Creator. And although we don't get to choose the body we want, we are responsible to take care of it! This journal will teach you how to honor your gift since it's the only one you'll ever receive. No matter what your current physical condition is, you can accomplish your goals with determination and persistence and time. Even though the majority of us weren't created with the "perfect" body, most of us would do amazingly well if we adopt the proper diet, the Transformetrics™ Training System, and journaling.

WHY JOURNALING IS INTEGRAL TO YOUR SUCCESS

Everything we know about the human race comes to us through recorded history. Etchings on the inside of caves show that even prehistoric people attempted to record significant events in their lives. One of the major differences between humanity and the animal kingdom is the fact that we have a written language that allows us to record our lives. And it is from our written records that we learn valuable lessons that help us to progress.

Perhaps you feel that diaries and journals seem a little tedious. I used to think they were a waste of time until I experimented with using a journal through the 60-day time frame. I found that not only could I record my fitness progress along with my eating habits, but it was interesting to watch how many patterns fluctuated due to what was going on in my life. Tracking my workout and eating habits inspire me to push harder, and it gives me confidence and a feeling of accomplishment. It's fun to go back and look at the progress you've made in the months and years past.

Journaling allows us to document and analyze the events that comprise our lives with objectivity and clarity, and it helps us remember. Our written records allow us to learn from the past and to shape our future with that knowledge. That's why Wendie and I are so adamant about keeping a written record, because *the best way to predict your future is to create it.*

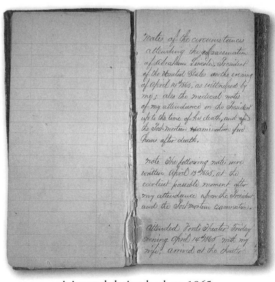

A journal dating back to 1865.

IDENTIFY REALISTIC GOALS
WEEK BY WEEK

There will be no "weigh days" in this journal—zero. The scale tells you a story that isn't worth listening to, and you should rather listen to what is important. How you feel, how your clothes fit, and, most importantly, your mental state are all stories that should be motivational as your fitness guide. You might be surprised at how your emotions can trigger unhealthy eating patterns and leave you with little or no desire to work out. Learn what triggers your eating—is it depression, boredom, anger, or are you a social eater? Once you learn what jump-starts your bad eating habits or discourages your intent to work out, you are more aware and will refrain from indulging your emotions.

If you identify a realistic goal each week as opposed to each month, your goal will be far more attainable. If you are out of shape and overweight, remember that you didn't get where you are overnight, and you won't get back to where you want to be overnight either—not safely anyway. Most people have let their bodies go for years, and then when they decide they're ready to lose weight and get in shape, they want it to happen instantly. But it just doesn't work that way. Losing 50 pounds in a month is not healthy, no matter how great it sounds. You need to set realistic goals to accomplish permanent weight-loss results.

Keep in mind that not all goals have to involve numbers. A realistic goal for you might be to eat fewer desserts, or to take the stairs instead of the elevator, or to try a new and fun cardio workout such as rollerblading or hiking. Pushing yourself every now and then will challenge you to make new goals.

This is your journal, so make as few or as many notes along the way that will help you progress in the future. Eventually, you'll create your own notes/short-hand system that makes it easier to log and read. Don't forget to choose periods of rest in between workout days. This will vary for everyone depending on their goals and how their bodies respond to each workout.

MY PERSONAL HISTORY

1 Describe your physical condition today:

_____
_____
_____
_____
_____
_____

2 What are your weaknesses as regards your physical condition?

_____
_____
_____
_____
_____
_____

3 What are your strengths? What has worked for you in the past?

_____
_____
_____
_____
_____
_____
_____

MY GOALS FOR THE
NEXT 60 DAYS

1 Regarding my physical condition, I want to:

_____

_____

_____

_____

_____

_____

2 I purpose to reach these goals by:

_____

_____

_____

_____

_____

_____

_____

3 I want to look and feel different in the following way:

_____

_____

_____

_____

_____

_____

_____

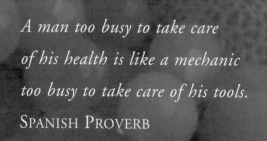

A man too busy to take care
of his health is like a mechanic
too busy to take care of his tools.
SPANISH PROVERB

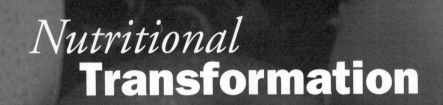

Nutritional **Transformation**

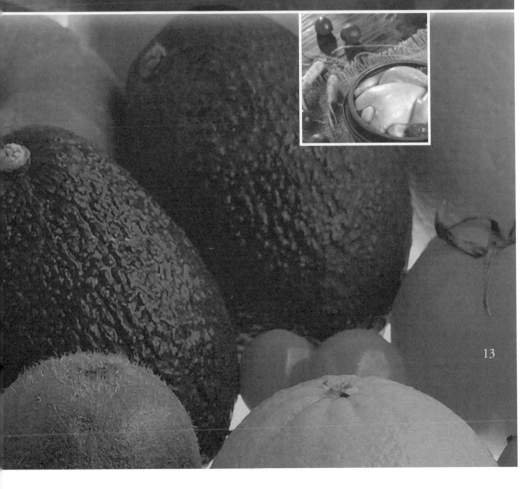

13

NUTRITIONAL TRANSFORMATION

1. *Awareness.* From now on it's important that you are aware of the nutritional value of the foods you choose to eat. In general, if you avoid eating foods that are processed and contain high concentrations of sugar and fat, you take a huge step toward achieving a lean, sculpted body.

2. *Self-Control.* From now on you will eat only until you are satisfied and not until you are full. For many people this requires a complete reeducation of personal nutrition habits. But once you are aware of this distinction you will be on your way to the lean, muscular physique you have always wanted.

3. *Question.* When dining out don't be afraid to be specific when asking your server about what a particular dish contains or how it is prepared. Learn to identify the hidden fat terms. "Lightly breaded" may mean "submerged in a tub of butter." Doing so can help you avoid hidden calories. And don't be afraid to ask for special preparations of menu items to reduce the fat.

4. *Be Consistent.* Several small meals as opposed to three large meals a day allow your body to process the food you eat much more efficiently while avoiding hunger or overeating at any given time.

5. *Hydrate Yourself* by drinking pure water. Depending upon your size, you'll need to drink at least 2 to 4 liters per day to obtain maximum benefit.

6. *Supplement Your Diet.* Because of the quality of our foods, it's difficult to get all the vitamins and minerals your body needs from the foods you eat. At the minimum, supplement your diet with a good food-based multivitamin to ensure you get all the nutrients you need.

7. *Refrain* from eating the wrong foods or at the wrong times. Your goal is to fuel your body with the best possible nutrients.

Let's Start Right...

Our goal is to change the ratio of lean muscle mass to stored body fat. But that does not necessarily mean "losing weight." In fact, I've worked with many people who gain 5 to 10 pounds of muscle while dropping inches from their waistline, hips, or buttocks. So don't concern yourself with what the scale says. In truth, all a scale does is measure the gravitational pull your body exerts to good old planet Earth. It tells you nothing about body density or the ratio of lean muscle mass to stored body fat.

And don't for one moment believe those ridiculous ads that promise 10 pounds of "weight loss" over the course of a weekend. The only way that is possible is for you to take strong diuretics and lose water weight. Even if you did lose one or two pounds of fat by severely reducing your calorie intake, the rest of the loss would be water, and just as soon as you start rehydrating yourself the weight will come back on, but with an important difference. *If you lose weight by starving yourself, your body automatically slows down its metabolism (the rate at which your body consumes energy or calories).* When that happens, you literally set yourself up to store body fat at a much faster rate when you go back to normal food consumption. And the truth is, this could easily cause you to gain more fat than when you started...the exact opposite of the goal you want to achieve.

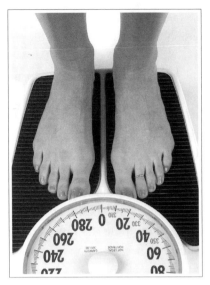

Lean, Strong, and Sculpted

Smart nutrition allows us to consume delicious, satisfying foods that provide our bodies with all it needs to maintain and build muscle tissue while simultaneously losing body fat. In fact, it is imperative that you eat enough high quality food and take high quality nutritional supplements in order to gain the most benefit from the Transformetrics™ Training System. The solution is simple: *Eat the right food at the right time, and your body will become a finely tuned fat-burning machine that will make you leaner and healthier overall.*

There is no *dieting* or *diet* involved. Instead, what Wendie and I are presenting is a positive lifestyle change. The bonus for implementing these changes includes not only a well-defined muscular physique but greatly improved health. Your cholesterol level will go down along with your blood pressure, while your energy level goes up. And this will happen *without* the sacrifice of delicious food. The only foods you will be giving up are unhealthy combinations of refined fats and carbohydrates (sugars). But before you learn how to eat for a lean, muscular, and sculpted look, take a quick course on the basics of good nutrition.

Calories

We've all heard or read the term *calories*. For instance, a 20-ounce bottle of Coca-Cola has 250 calories, according to the nutritional information on the label (which you need to check regularly). Why is that a big deal? Isn't a calorie just a calorie, after all? No. You need to look closer. According to the label, those 250 calories are comprised solely of sugar (carbohydrates)—*more than 60 grams of sugar!* More on that later.

Here's what you need to understand about food consumption. A calorie is simply a unit that measures the amount of energy required to raise the temperature of a gram of water by 1°C. All food contains energy (calories) or potential fuel for the body to operate and perform its many functions. Not unlike a car that will not operate without proper fuel, your body will not function properly if you don't eat. In fact, given enough time and a complete lack of food (fuel), your body will eventually starve to death. However, although an intake of "good" calories is absolutely essential for strength and fitness, not all calories are of equal value, and there are some calories you would be better off to avoid completely.

Here's why you need to discriminate in your calorie intake. The food you eat is divided into three basic categories—fats, proteins, and carbohydrates. Of the three, fats contain more than twice the number of calories per gram of either protein or carbohydrates. A gram of fat contains 9 calories whereas a gram of carbohydrate or protein supplies only 4 calories. In other words, 1 gram of fat at 9 calories contains more calories than 1 gram of protein and 1 gram of carbohydrate combined, which together equals only 8 calories.

But that's not the end of the "fatness" of fat calories. In one sense, fat calories really go straight to the waistline. This is true because it takes little or no energy for your body to digest fats. Only about 3 percent of the energy created by fat calories is used in the digestion process. This is also true with refined sugars. By comparison, it takes a great deal more energy to digest either protein or unrefined complex carbohydrate calories. In fact, laboratory studies have proven that it requires about 15 percent of the calories from either proteins or unrefined complex carbohydrates just to complete the digestion process. Simply put, when you consume fat or sugars (refined carbohydrates), you're feeding your body calories that require almost no digestion at all. And since most of us don't make our living by climbing mountains, these refined calories are immediately available for storage at their favorite fat storage sites on your body. This is not a good thing.

Protein

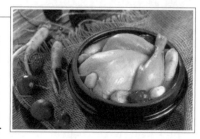

Unless you've been living in a cave for the last few years, you're aware that protein is your friend in the quest for a lithe, muscular, sculpted body. And Wendie and I don't dispute this because it's absolutely true—especially when you consider that most of your body material is composed of protein! Muscle, internal organs, blood, hair, and even your fingernails are all composed of protein. In addition, protein also plays a major role in regulating water balance throughout your body. Important? You bet.

First, we need to define protein. Protein are large, complex molecules composed of 22 amino acids. Eight of the amino acids are produced by the human body, but the other 14 "essential amino acids" are not and must be obtained from foods that contain them. The foods that contain all 14 essential amino acids are red meats, poultry, fish, milk and milk products, and eggs. The problem with relying solely on these sources of complete protein is that some of these products are also very high in fat (with the exception of egg whites).

So although these foods are excellent sources of protein, we recommend that you obtain your protein requirements for the most part from low-fat sources, such as the white meat of chickens and turkeys, ultra lean meats such as wild game, buffalo, and lamb, fish of all types, low-fat dairy products, and egg whites. In addition, there are exceptional protein supplements readily available at local health food stores that offer the highest possible protein efficiency ratios (or PER) and at relatively inexpensive prices, especially when compared to expensive cuts of meat and fish. The bottom line is that obtaining good lean protein sources is easier today than it has ever been. So rest assured you'll be able to feed your muscles and body tissues everything they need without breaking your bank account to do it.

Protein Requirements

So how much protein does your body need? According to scientific research, the human body can only absorb 30 to 40 grams of protein at any given time. Hence our recommendation to eat 5 to 6 small meals daily as opposed to 2 or 3 large meals. It's much easier on the body's digestion, and it allows for much more of the protein you consume to be utilized in body maintenance and muscle building. Over consumption of protein, at any given time, will either be stored as body fat or excreted from the body, causing a strain on the digestive system, and neither one is healthy option. Ideally, eat 5 to 6 small meals daily as opposed to 2 or 3 large meals.

Carbohydrates

During the 1990s, nutritional scientists (funded by the food processors) told people to avoid protein and all forms of *fat*—even the essential fatty acids that are necessary for life and normal cell function not to mention the body's ability to synthesize hormones. As a result of following these so-called dietary experts, diabetes and obesity skyrocketed to epidemic proportions. So much so that today an uninformed public is frightened to eat carbohydrates. *But carbs are not to blame!* As usual, misinformation is.

Here's how it worked. During the '90s, while we were bombarded with constant messages on television and in the print media about the dangers of fat, we were simultaneously blitzed with messages from food manufacturers telling us to eat their low-fat cakes, brownies, and cookies. What they neglected to tell us was that these processed products were super high in refined sugars and appetite-stimulating chemical additives that made people lose control over their appetites, thereby causing them to consume twice as many calories as they otherwise would have. To make matters worse, these products had almost no dietary fiber. America's consumption of these foods led to rampant obesity and diabetes nationwide. And what was blamed? You guessed it—carbohydrates.

Just as the right amount of proteins and fats is absolutely essential for health and overall well-being, so are carbohydrates. In fact, if you starve your body by not fueling it with the right kind of carbohydrates, you'll get to the point where you can't even think straight and you'll feel edgy all the time. But it's the right kind of carbohydrates that are essential to good health.

There are three types of carbohydrates: refined (manufactured by man); simple (natural occurring sugars created by God and found in an abundance of natural fruits); and complex (found in grains and vegetables of all types). Let's look at them individually.

Refined Carbohydrates

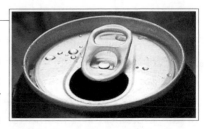

These are man-made sugars. Remember when I previously referred to that 20-ounce bottle of Coke? On the label it stated that it contained 250 calories and 60+ grams of sugar. No protein, no fat, no vitamins, no minerals (other than phosphoric acid which will destroy your skeletal tissues, muscles, bones, and connective tissue over time). Did I mention no fiber, but it does have caffeine and food coloring? That's it, folks. In other words, it has nothing but ultra-refined carbohydrates that require virtually no digestion, that go right into your bloodstream and cause an insulin spike, so that just as you feel a rush of energy, it's followed by an even bigger letdown. Then after these ultra-refined carbs have entered your bloodstream, where would you guess those 250 calories go if you don't burn them off in activity? Look down at your waist, because you'll be wearing them in body fat.

This is why refined sugars are so bad for you. They have been stripped of all life-giving nutrients, including vitamins, minerals, and dietary fiber. As a result, they can be immediately stored on the body. But also consider this: If sugar can be responsible for literally eating holes in tooth enamel, the hardest structure of your body, what else can it do? Bottom line: If you want to be strong and super healthy, it's essential to keep ultra-refined sugars (carbohydrates) to a minimum and consume them very infrequently. Does that mean never? Of course not. Even Charles Atlas said it was okay to eat sweets once in a while, provided that it was of the highest quality possible.

Simple Carbohydrates

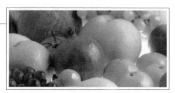

These are the naturally occurring sugars found in an abundance of delicious fruits. The good news is that in the form provided by nature, you also get vitamins, minerals, water, and phytonutrients that are completely absent from processed, man-made refined sugars. So if you want to indulge in a dietary treat that's good for you, it's essential that you include an abundance of fresh fruits. Sweets as God intended.

Complex Carbohydrates

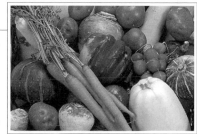

Complex carbohydrates come in the form of grains and vegetables. The molecular structure of these carbohydrates requires a gradual break-down into glucose, which results in slowly released energy over a much larger period of time (up to 4 hours) than simple carbohydrates or the refined, man-made version. For this reason vegetables (fresh, frozen, and canned) and whole grains should become your dietary mainstay with unprocessed simple carbohydrates (fruits) as your backup, and keep the ultra-refined carbohydrates as your binge-avoiding treat. Complex carbohydrates in their unrefined state give you plenty of dietary fiber and allow your appetite to feel satiated for longer periods of time. Yams, squash, potatoes, carrots, and virtually all whole grains, including rice, corn, oats, wheat, rye, and several others, offer incredible health benefits in helping to control cholesterol and improve your overall triglyceride profile.

Bottom line: Don't be afraid to eat unrefined carbohydrates as nature intended them. But do yourself a favor. Avoid all *refined* carbohydrates that are high in sugars and fats, such as pies, cookies, cakes, ice cream, potato chips, and all refined snack foods. These are the foods (if you want to call them that) that are responsible for both the obesity and diabetes epidemics in America today. The food processors would rather die than admit it, but that doesn't make it any less true.

Sodium—The Truth

Sodium, in combination with potassium, helps regulate body fluids and maintain the acid-alkali balance of the bloodstream. This sodium-potassium balance is necessary for many bodily functions, not the least of which is the ability of muscles to contract. This is why certain athletes develop cramps in the latter part of intense competitions when they have been sweating so much that this delicate balance becomes disrupted. Such episodes have cost many athletes world titles as happened to Muhammad Ali when he fought Leon Spinks the first time. He literally couldn't protect himself because he became so weak. In addition to losing the ability to control and contract muscles, insufficient sodium can also cause muscle shrinking and intestinal gas.

For this reason, it is not necessary for healthy people to completely eliminate sodium from their diet. And in any case, it would be very difficult to do because virtually everything we eat and drink contains some sodium. Tap water contains 10 milligrams of sodium in an 8-ounce glass. Club soda contains 25 milligrams per 8-ounce serving as do virtually all soft drinks. Even a slice of whole wheat bread contains 120 milligrams while a 6-ounce chicken breast contains 150 milligrams. So you see it really isn't difficult to obtain reasonable amounts of sodium.

So why is sodium considered to be so bad? Simple. Sodium holds up to 50 times its own weight in water. Excess sodium consumption results in water retention. In fact, it is not unusual for many people to carry 5 to 10 pounds of excess water in their bodies if they habitually consume extremely high sodium foods. This in turn can lead to problems such as high blood pressure.

Balance

Although Wendie and I do not believe it is necessary for a healthy person to totally deprive themselves of sodium, too much can cause all kinds of problems. So what we recommend is that you strive to stay between 1,500 and 2,500 milligrams daily. Foods that contain excessive amounts of sodium include all canned, smoked, and pickled foods, most frozen dinners, Chinese foods, pizza, frankfurters, and condiments such as table salt, ketchup, mustard, A-1 sauce, and Worcestershire sauce. These items can easily contain 1,000 or more milligrams per serving, so go easy on these.

If you are one of the very few people who enjoys high sodium foods and has no problem with high blood pressure, and if you don't mind the temporary water weight gain obscuring the muscular definition of your abdominals and other muscle groups, it's probably not a big deal to indulge in pizza once in a while. All you need to do is to cut way back for a period of 3 to 5 days on sodium intake and drink lots of pure H_2O, and you'll eliminate any excess water and find that no real harm has been done.

Remember, water weight is not *real* weight. It's very temporary and can be flushed out of your system in a matter of days. Fat weight, on the other hand, is all *too real*. It sticks to your muscles and takes weeks to eliminate. But it too will go away.

Drink Lots of Water

Isn't it ironic that the best way to get rid of excess water weight is to drink more of it? It's true. The more water you drink, the less water you retain. You will also retain less water while eating high sodium foods if you drink a lot of water while eating. Drink a minimum of eight 12-ounce glasses of pure water daily. It's a great way to keep your skin looking younger and also gives your body a daily internal shower.

The Lean, Sculpted, Muscular Food Plan

Now that you know the basics about food, it's time to plan your new healthy eating style. The quintessence (I've always wanted to use that word) of the plan is simple. Wendie has compiled a Five Tier List of the best foods for getting lean, sculpted, and muscular on the hurry up. Starting with List One—"Best Foods to Get 'Ripped By' "—read all the way down through List Five—"Eat This Stuff Often and You'll Be Wearing It."

You'll have a complete and ready reference to review anytime and anyplace. Best of all is the fact that if 80 percent of your food choices come from Lists One and Two, 15 percent come from List Three, and only 5 percent coming from Lists Four and Five, you will be awed by how easy it is to stay lean, hard, and sculpted. So here are the lists, the rest is up to you.

Good Luck!

FOOD LISTS	%
LISTS ONE & TWO	80%
LIST THREE	15%
LISTS FOUR & FIVE	5%

PERSONAL POWER FOOD PLANNER
for the Lean, Sculpted, Muscular Look

LIST ONE
BEST FOODS TO GET "RIPPED BY"

- Artichokes
- Beans, all varieties
- Bee pollen, organic
- Beets
- Blackberries
- Blueberries
- Boysenberries
- Bran
- **BROCCOLI**
- Brussels sprouts
- Cabbage
- Cantaloupe
- Carrots
- Cauliflower
- Cereals, whole grain only
- Citrus, raw fruits & juices w/no sugar added
- Cranberry juice, all natural
- Currants
- Eggs, poached
- Fish, cold water varieties (salmon, mackerel, cod)
- Garlic, fresh
- Grapes and grape juice, no added sugar
- Kale
- **KIWI FRUIT**
- Mangoes

- Milk, nonfat
- Mushrooms (portabello, miiake, and shitake)
- Nectarines
- Oatmeal, steel cut
- Olives
- Olive oil
- Onions
- **PAPAYAS**
- Peas
- Peppers, red and green
- Plums
- Protein drinks, whey protein low fat/low sugar
- Prunes
- Rice, brown
- Salsa
- Spinach, fresh
- Sweet potatoes
- Tea, green and black
- Tofu
- Tomatoes and tomato products
- Vegetable juices, fresh squeezed
- Water

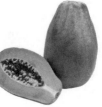
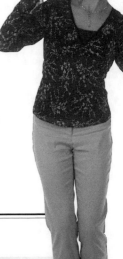

EXCEPTIONAL FOODS FOR HEALTH & STRENGTH

- Almonds, raw
- Apples
- Asparagus
- **BANANAS**
- Barley
- Boca burgers
- Bread, sprouted whole grain
- Broccoli sprouts
- Buffalo steaks (lower in fat than chicken)
- Celery
- Cereal, dry, high-fiber varieties
- Cherries, fresh, all varieties
- Chicken, free range, skinless white meat
- Coffee, black
- Cottage cheese, low fat
- **CORN ON THE COB**
- Cucumbers
- Eggplant
- Goat's milk
- Fish, fresh water varieties
- Graham crackers
- Lettuce, romaine, leafy green, or red
- Lima beans
- Melon, honeydew
- Mushrooms (morels)
- Ostrich
- Pancakes, buckwheat

- Pasta, high protein, with marinara sauce, fish, or vegetables
- Peaches
- Pears
- Pecans
- **PINEAPPLE**
- Raisins
- Raspberries
- Rhubarb
- Ricotta cheese
- Shellfish, boiled or broiled
- Soy beans, edemame
- Soy milk
- Squash, butternut and summer
- Strawberries
- String beans
- Sunflower seeds
- Tuna, albacore packed in spring water
- Turkey breast
- Vegetable juice, canned or bottled
- Veggie burgers
- Walnuts
- **WATERMELON**
- Wine, red
- Yogurt, low-fat varieties
- Zucchini

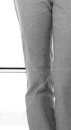
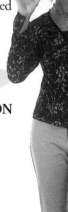

GREAT FOOD! BUT USE LISTS ONE & TWO FOR RAPID FAT LOSS

- Applesauce
- Apricots
- **AVOCADOS**
- Bagels, whole grain
- Beef, eye of round
- Beef, extra lean ground
- Beef, London broil
- Beef, top round
- Canola oil
- Chicken, broiled
- Chicken taco, baked
- Chicken wrap, white meat
- Chocolate, dark natural
- Eggs, whole
- English muffins, whole grain
- French fries, baked
- Fruit, dried
- Fruit juice, unsweetened
- Granola, natural low fat
- Iced coffee and tea drinks with nonfat milk
- Jams and marmalade, all-natural fruit
- **LAMB, ROAST LEG**

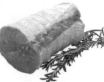

- Margarine, fat free
- Mustard
- Nuts (walnuts, macadamia, pastachios, hazelnuts, pine nuts)
- Olives
- Pancakes
- Pasta, plain
- Peanut oil
- **PEANUTS**
- Peanut butter, all natural
- Pork tenderloin
- Potatoes, white
- Pretzels, whole grain
- Refried beans, low fat
- Rice cakes
- Rice, long grain basmati
- Sauerkraut
- Soups, canned broth
- Veal, roasted
- Wine, white
- Yogurt with natural fruit

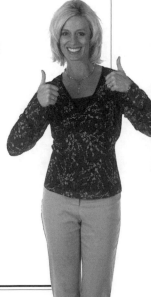

BE CAREFUL! STILL, ONCE IN A WHILE IS NO BIG DEAL

- Beef (barbecued, filet mignon, rib eye, sirloin)
- **BEEF, LEAN GROUND**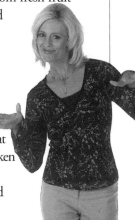
- Beef stroganoff with fat-free sour cream
- Butter
- Caesar salad with chicken
- Canadian bacon
- Cheese, natural varieties only
- Chili
- Chinese food with lots of vegetables
- Chips, baked, low fat, whole grain
- **COFFEE CAKE**
- Crackers, whole grain
- Cream cheese, low fat
- Duck, roasted
- Energy bars, whole grain
- Fruits, canned in natural juices
- Grilled cheese sandwich, natural cheeses only
- Ham, ultra lean
- Honey
- Hot dogs, low fat
- Lettuce, iceberg
- Juices, sweetened w/pear juice
- Lamb chops
- Lasagna, low-fat meat or vegetable
- Lunch meat, deli style lean
- Macaroni and cheese
- Macaroni salad
- Mayonnaise, low fat
- Meat loaf
- Mexican food, not fried
- Milk, 2% butterfat
- Muffins
- Nut butters (almond/cashew)
- Peppers, stuffed
- **PIZZA**
- Popcorn w/butter
- Pork chops, ultra lea
- Potato salad
- Pudding, low fat
- Reuben sandwich or wrap
- Salads (chef's, chicken, cobb, tuna)
- Sherbet
- Sloppy Joe, ultra lean
- Sorbet made from fresh fruit
- Soups, creamed varieties
- Soy sauce
- Spaghetti with meatballs
- Submarine sandwich, ultra lean, low fat
- Taco salad, chicken or lean beef
- Turkey, ground
- Vegetable oils, cold processed

EAT THIS STUFF OFTEN AND YOU'LL BE WEARING IT!

- Bacon
- Beef, ground, regular
- Beef tacos, deep fried
- Breakfast sandwiches, fast food varieties
- **CAKES**
- Candies
- Cereals, pre-sugared
- Charred or blackened beef, chicken, or fish
- Cheese curds, deep fried
- Chicken divan
- Chicken nuggets
- Chicken wings, buffalo or sweet and sour
- Chicken sandwich, fried
- Chips, potato or corn, industrial strength regular
- Cinnamon buns, glazed
- Clams
- Clam chowder
- **COOKIES**
- Corn dogs
- Crab
- Cream cheese
- Creamed vegetables
- Creamer, nondairy
- Doughnuts, all varieties
- French fries
- Gravies
- Hamburger, fast food
- Hot dogs
- Ice cream, full-fat varieties
- Latte with whole milk
- Lobster Newburg
- Lunchmeat
- Mayonnaise, industrial strength
- Milk, whole
- Nacho chips with cheese
- Onion rings
- Pastries
- **PIES**
- Potatoes, fried
- Potato skins with standard toppings
- Pot pies
- Refried beans, the real ones in lard
- Salad dressings, full-fat varieties
- Sausages
- Shrimp, breaded and fried
- Soft drinks
- Spare ribs
- Tater tots
- Toaster pastries

There you have it. Follow this five tier list and it will be easy to stay in lean, well-muscled condition 24/7.

If you mess up once in a while, no big deal. Just concentrate on lists one, two, and three until you're back to lean.

Now let's look at some serious body sculpting from neck to toes!

TAKE CONTROL

What is it about seeing that last cookie in the cookie jar and the immediate feeling that we should just go ahead and eat it, yet after we gobble it down we feel guilty? Or how about eating the last handful of chips in the bag that was left over from a neighborhood party. Certainly, there are times when you will have foods in your house that aren't on your eating plan, such as having company or parties. But once they leave and the party is over, find something else to do with the leftover junk food besides eating it! I assure you that you won't hurt the food's feelings!

If disposing of junk food seems like commonsense to you, you may be in the minority. Take a look around your friend's pantry or refrigerator and see what kinds of foods are lingering. You'll typically find eating environments that are disorderly. For that matter, take a look around your own eating environment. What's there?

If you feel guilty about throwing out foods that you know you shouldn't eat, I understand. Most of us have had it drilled into us that we should never waste food. Below is a list of ways to incorporate good eating habits and ways to simplify your environment to leap to "a brand new you!"

• Send food home with your party guests or take the leftovers to work. Anything to get it out of the house is key to your health and fitness success.

• Dispose of all high-calorie, high-fat foods from your house. Your first line of defense is to keep these foods out of your reach.

• Do yourself a big favor and keep all-natural healthy foods in sight.

• Drink a 12- or 16-ounce glass of water before a meal.

• Don't go to the grocery store hungry. Plan a one- to two-week shopping list so you don't have to go back and forth to the store. Better yet, online shopping will keep you from being tempted to reach for something you don't need.

• Eat slowly and take breaks while eating. It takes an average of 20 to 30 minutes for the brain to tell you that you're full.

• Cook without fat. Grill, bake, or broil instead.

• Portion sizes should be considered. Remember the rule: the palm of your hand is an adequate serving size.

- Use a smaller plate.

- Limit desserts. If you must "clean your palate," then make the dessert light, or better yet, eat a small piece of fruit.

- Stay away from any product that has trans fats.

- Don't serve or go to restaurants that serve "family style."

- Don't be afraid to ask the waiter at a restaurant to eliminate butter, oils, etc. that may make the meal high in calories. Once you are satisfied with your meal, stop eating. Don't keep looking at whatever is left on your plate or you will eat it. Ask the waiter to take it away.

- Use skim milk whenever possible.

- As much as possible, don't eat after 7 p.m. The later you eat, the less chance you have of burning up the calories.

- Take photos of yourself every two weeks.

Once you start eliminating some of your bad habits, you will be on the road to success. This journal will help you recognize your negative patterns so they may be corrected with positive choices. It's amazing how just a few small changes can make a huge impact to get you motivated, enabling you to reach your fitness goals. Keep your journal handy so that recording is easy and painless. This journal will be one of the keys to your fitness success. You can only enhance what God gave you!

THE GLYCEMIC INDEX

The Glycemic Index is just one of the many tools you have available to help improve your dietary control. Complex carbohydrates burn more slowly and, for the most part, help regulate the amount of sugar released into the bloodstream. The rate at which blood sugar levels rise after a specific food is eaten is called its glycemic index, which was devised as a means to help diabetics in their food selections. One of the values of this general index is that it shows that even among carbohydrates, there is a wide range of variance of values. For instance, the potato is actually a high-glycemic food that can spike one's insulin levels and should be eaten in moderation.

The numbers below are based on glucose, which is the fastest carbohydrate available except for maltose. *Glucose is given a value of 100—other carbs are given a number relative to glucose.* Any glycemic value over 50 (other experts say 60) is considered to be high (that's one-half the value of glucose). Faster carbs (higher numbers) are great for raising low blood sugars and for covering brief periods of intense exercise. Slower carbs (lower numbers) are helpful for preventing overnight drops in the blood sugar and for long periods of exercise.

These numbers are compiled from a wide range of research labs, and as often as possible from more than one study. These numbers will be close but may not be identical to other glycemic index lists. The impact a food will have on blood sugars depends on many other factors, such as ripeness, cooking time, fiber and fat content, time of day, blood insulin levels, and recent activity.

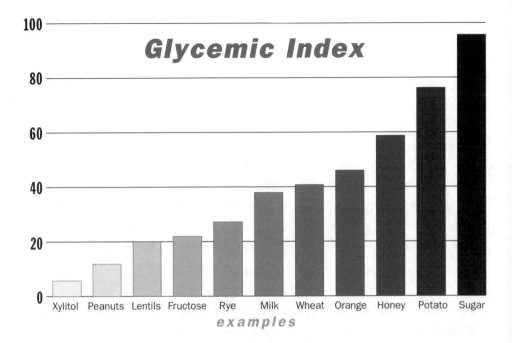

Glycemic Index

Xylitol · Peanuts · Lentils · Fructose · Rye · Milk · Wheat · Orange · Honey · Potato · Sugar

examples

GLYCEMIC REFERENCE LIST

Beans

baby lima **32**
baked **43**
black **30**
brown **38**
butter **31**
chickpeas **33**
kidney **27**
lentil **30**
navy **38**
pinto **42**
red lentils **27**
split peas **32**
soy **18**

Breads

bagel **72**
croissant **67**
kaiser roll **73**
pita **57**
pumpernickel **49**
rye **64**
rye, dark **76**
rye, whole **50**
white **72**
whole wheat **72**

Cereals

All Bran **44**
Bran Chex **58**
Cheerios **74**
Corn Bran **75**
Corn Chex **83**
Cornflakes **83**
Cream of Wheat **66**
Crispix **87**
Frosted Flakes **55**
Grapenuts **67**
Grapenuts Flakes **80**
Life **66**
Muesli **60**
NutriGrain **66**
Oatmeal **49**
Oatmeal 1 min **66**
Puffed Wheat **74**

Puffed Rice **90**
Rice Bran **19**
Rice Chex **89**
Rice Krispies **82**
Shredded Wheat **69**
Special K **54**
Swiss Muesli **60**
Total **76**

Cookies

Graham crackers **74**
oatmeal **55**
shortbread **64**
Vanilla Wafers **77**

Crackers

rice cakes **82**
rye **63**
saltine **72**
stoned wheat thins **67**
water crackers **78**

Desserts

angel food cake **67**
banana bread **47**
blueberry muffin **59**
bran muffin **60**
Danish **59**
fruit bread **47**
pound cake **54**
sponge cake **46**

Fruit

apple **38**
apricot, canned **64**
apricot, dried **30**
banana **62**
banana, unripe **30**
cantaloupe **65**
cherries **22**
dates, dried **103**
fruit cocktail **55**
grapefruit **25**
grapes **43**
kiwi **52**
mango **55**
orange **43**
papaya **58**
peach **42**
pear **36**
pineapple **66**
plum **24**
raisins **64**
strawberries **32**
strawberry jam **51**
watermelon **72**

Grains

barley **22**
brown rice **59**
buckwheat **54**
bulgur **47**
chickpeas **36**
cornmeal **68**
couscous **65**
hominy **40**
millet **75**
rice, instant **91**
rice, parboiled **47**
rye **34**
sweet corn **55**
wheat, whole **41**
white rice **88**

Juices

agave nectar **11**
apple **41**
grapefruit **48**
orange **55**
pineapple **46**

Milk Products

ice cream **50**
milk **34**
pudding **43**
soy milk **31**
yogurt **38**

Pasta

brown rice pasta **92**
gnocchi **68**
linguine, durum **50**
macaroni **46**
macaroni and cheese **64**
spaghetti **40**

vermicelli **35**
vermicelli, rice **58**

Sweets

honey **58**
jelly beans **80**
Life Savers **70**
M&M's Chocolate peanuts **33**
Skittles **70**
Snickers **41**

Vegetables

beets **70**
carrots **85**
corn **70–85**
green peas **51**
green vegetables **0–15**
onions **10**
parsnips **95**
potatoes, new **58**
potatoes, russet **98**
potatoes, sweet **50**
potatoes, white **70–90**
pumpkin **75**
rutabaga **71**

GO FOR THE FIBER!

Fiber comes from the cell walls and other parts of plants, with fresh, live foods being the best source. It is a key to a low glycemic diet and essential for good health. A diet rich in fiber can help fight obesity, heart disease, diabetes, and cancer. It slows down the digestive process and helps regulate the release of insulin into the bloodstream, which allows for a steady supply of energy over a longer period of time. Beyond that, fiber gives you that "full" feeling and then speeds the transit time of fecal matter out of the body, which makes it highly valuable.

While Americans eat an average of 12–17 grams of fiber daily, the American Dietetic Association recommends an intake of 20–25 grams, and some experts say that for optimal health a person should get 40–60 grams a day.

Fiber comes in two forms: soluble and insoluble. Soluble fiber, which is present in legumes, brans, fruits, vegetable, whole grain products, seeds and nuts, and psyllium seed, helps to reduce cholesterol and to balance blood sugar levels. Insoluble fiber, found in whole wheat products, brown rice, kidney beans, skins of fruits, and many vegetables, reduce the risk of constipation as well as help prevent bowel cancer.

Good fiber, for instance, is found in a bowl of oat bran and fresh fruit. A pathetic attempt is a bran muffin loaded with processed sugars and preservatives.

A SAMPLE OF FIBER CONTENT OF FOODS

(fiber value is in grams)

fiber value	
14.7	Almonds (slivered, dried, 1 cup)
3.0	Apple (small, with skin)
4.7	Avocado (1 whole)
0	Bacon
10.0	Beans, kidney (½ cup)
8.2	Beans, sprouts (½ cup)
10.5	Bran, oat (½ cup)
15.6	Bran, wheat (½ cup)
2.78	Carrots (chopped, ½ cup)
6.0	Cornmeal (stone ground, ½ cup)
0	Doughnuts
7.5	Figs (dried, chopped, ½ cup)
3.4	Flour, all-purpose white (1 cup)
13.0	Flour, whole wheat (1 cup)
7.8	Lentils (cooked, ½ cup)
0.7	Lettuce, romaine (shredded, ½ cup)
0	Meat
6.3	Pasta, whole wheat (1 cup)
4.6	Pear (1 medium)
0.9	Pepper, green (1 large)
2.1	Potato, white (2.25" diameter)
16.1	Prunes, dried (8 large)
5.4	Raisins (½ cup)
6.4	Raspberries (½ cup)
4.2	Rice, brown (½ cup)
9.6	Soybeans (½ cup)
0.15	Spaghetti, white (½ cup)
1.7	Strawberries (½ cup)

VITAMIN AND MINERAL SUPPLEMENTATION

*V*itamins constitute one of the major groups of nutrients, which are food substances necessary for growth and health. They regulate chemical reactions through which the body converts food into energy and living tissues. Thus they have a key role in producing energy for each and every cell in the body. Vitamins also help to manufacture enzymes, which do wide-ranging tasks within the body from digesting food to making neurotransmitters. Of the 13 vitamins we need, 5 are produced by the body itself. Of those 5, only 3 can be produced in sufficient quantities to meet the body's needs. Therefore, vitamins must be supplied in a person's daily diet.

We tend to think that any vitamin will do, but this is not the case. Every vitamin has a specific function that nothing else can replace. And, if you lack any vitamin, it can actually hinder the function of another. Vitamin deficiency diseases, such as beriberi, pellagra, rickets, or scurvy, are the result of an ongoing lack of a vitamin.

A well-balanced diet from all the basic food groups is the best way to obtain these essential vitamins. If you take supplements, always take a food-based multivitamin capsule as well as specific nutrients to help them work more effectively. Do not exceed the doses printed on the packaging.

Minerals are nutrients that function alongside of vitamins as components of body enzymes. While they are needed in small amounts, they are absolutely essential for the biochemical processes of the body to work. Without your minerals in adequate supply, you can't absorb the vitamins. Minerals are needed for proper composition of teeth and bone and blood and muscle and nerve cells. They are important to the production of hormones and enzymes and in the creation of antibodies. Some minerals (calcium, potassium, and sodium) have electrical charges that act as a magnet to attract other electrically charged substances to form complex molecules, conduct electrical impulses (messages) along nerves, and transport substances in and out of the cells. Magnesium and manganese are essential to convert carbohydrates into energy for the brain.

DAILY OPTIMAL VITAMIN AND MINERAL SUPPLEMENTATION

The following recommendations for daily intake levels of vitamins and minerals are designed to provide an optimum intake range for maintaining good health. If possible, buy natural, organic vitamins, preferably labeled as not having sugar, preservatives, lactose, yeast, or starch. Also follow instructions regarding storage and recommended dosage. Some minerals and vitamins are toxic in high doses, and the safe dose can be exceeded if you take supplements from more than one source.

VITAMINS	SUPPLEMENTARY DOSAGE RANGE
Vitamin A (retinal)	5,000–10,000 IU
Vitamin A (from beta-carotene)	10,000–75,000 IU
Vitamin D	100–400 IU
Vitamin E (d-alpha tocopherol)	400–1,200 IU
Vitamin K (phytonadione)	60–900 mcg.
Vitamin C (ascorbic acid)	500–9,000 mg.
Vitamin B1 (thiamine)	10–90 mg.
Vitamin B2 (riboflavin)	10–90 mg.
Niacin	10–90 mg.
Niacin amide	10–30 mg.
Vitamin B6 (pyridoxine)	25–100 mg.
Biotin	100–300 mcg.
Pantothenic acid	25–100 mg.
Folic acid	400–1,000 mcg.
Vitamin B12	400–1,000 mcg.
Choline	150–500 mg.
Inositol	150–500 mg.

MINERALS	SUPPLEMENTARY DOSAGE RANGE
Boton	1–2 mg.
Calcium	250–750 mg.
Chromium	200–400 mcg.
Copper	1–2 mg.
Iodine	50–150 mcg.
Iron	15–30 mg.
Magnesium	250–750 mg.
Manganese (citrate)	10–15 mg.
Molybdenum (sodium molybdate)	10–25 mcg.
Potassium	200–500 mg.
Selenium (selenomethionine)	100–200 mcg.
Silica (sodium metasilicate)	200–1,000 mcg.
Vanadium (sulfate)	50–100 mcg.
Zinc (picolinate)	15–30 mcg.

HEALTHY SNACKS

Almonds

Applesauce

Avocado with a squeeze of lemon and ground pepper

Bananas

Banana flan pie

Blue chips

Carob brownies

Carob covered almonds

Carrot sticks

Celery sticks with almond butter

Cheese sticks (organic)

Chinese rice crackers

Cocoa

Dried fruits (organic)

Eggs, boiled

Granola bars

Granola with almonds

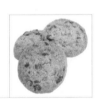

Kefir

Mineral tonic

Oatmeal raisin cookies

Raisins (organic)

Protein bars

100% rye crackers

Strawberries

Turkey jerky (organic)

Walnuts

Yogurt

Yogurt covered almonds

Yogurt parfait

Yogurt pie

JUNK FOOD

"Junk food" is a general term that has come to encompass foods that offer little in terms of protein, minerals, or vitamins, and lots of calories from sugar or fat. We're talking about high-sugar, low-fiber, and high-fat foods that attract us and our children like magnets and put enormous stress on our healing system.

While there is no definitive list of junk foods, most authorities include foods that are high in salt, sugar, or fat calories, and low nutrient content. The big hitters on most people's lists include fried fast food, salted snack foods, carbonated beverages, candies, gum, and most sweet desserts. The term "empty calories" reflects the lack of nutrients found in junk food.

According to a recent study in the *American Journal of Clinical Nutrition,* one-third of the average American's diet is made up of junk foods. Because junk foods take the place of healthier foods, these same Americans are depending on the other two-thirds of their diet to get 100 percent of the recommended dietary intake of vitamins and nutrients. Studies show that the average American gets 27 percent of their total daily energy from junk foods and an additional 4 percent from alcoholic beverages. About one-third of Americans consume an average of 45 percent of energy from these foods. Researchers are certain that such patterns of eating may have long-term, even life-threatening, health consequences.

If you have any question about the nutritional value of a food, judge it by the list of ingredients and the Nutrition Facts label found on packages. That label will list the number of calories per serving, grams of fat, sodium, cholesterol, fiber, and sugar content. If sugar, fat, or salt show up as one of the first three ingredients, you can probably consider that food to be a nutritional risk.

CHECK OUT THE FOOD LABEL

By law, most of the foods purchased today must carry a nutrition label. But food labels are more than just a federal requirement—once you understand the information they provide, you can use food labels as a guide to planning healthier meals and snacks. It's important that you understand what you're actually buying. Look at the "Nutrition Facts" on a product label for the specific information on such vital factors as nutrients, calories, total fat, saturated fat, cholesterol, sodium, total carbohydrates, dietary fiber as well as the serving size. As you consider the calorie and fat values, make sure you understand the serving size. You may be surprised by what you find is in what you were about to purchase.

The FDA also provides guidelines about the claims and descriptions manufacturers may use in food labeling to promote their products:

Claim Requirements That Must Be Met

Fat-Free
Less than 0.5 grams of fat per serving, with no added fat or oil

Low fat
3 grams or less of fat per serving

Less fat
25% or less fat than the comparison food

Saturated Fat Free
Less than 0.5 grams of saturated fat and 0.5 grams of trans fatty acids per serving

Cholesterol-Free
Less than 2 mg cholesterol per serving, and 2 grams or less saturated fat per serving

Low Cholesterol
20 mg or less cholesterol per serving and 2 grams or less saturated fat per serving

Reduced Calorie
At least 25% fewer calories per serving than the comparison food

Low Calorie
40 calories or less per serving

Claim Requirements That Must Be Met

Extra Lean
Less than 5 grams of fat, 2 grams of saturated fat, and 95 mg of cholesterol per (100 gram) serving of meat, poultry, or seafood

Lean
Less than 10 grams of fat, 4.5 g of saturated fat, and 95 mg of cholesterol per (100 gram) serving of meat, poultry, or seafood

Light (fat)
50% or less of the fat than in the comparison food (ex.: 50% less fat than our regular cheese)

Light (calories)
1/3 fewer calories than the comparison food

High-Fiber
5 grams or more fiber per serving

Sugar-Free
Less than 0.5 grams of sugar per serving

Sodium-Free
Less than 5 mg of sodium per serving

Low Sodium
140 mg or less per serving

Very Low Sodium
35 mg or less per serving

Healthy
A food low in fat, saturated fat, cholesterol, and sodium, and contains at least 10% of the Daily Values for vitamin A, vitamin C, iron, calcium, protein, or fiber.

"High," "Rich in," or "Excellent Source"
20% or more of the Daily Value for a given nutrient per serving

"Less," "Fewer," or "Reduced"
At least 25% less of a given nutrient or calories than the comparison food

"Low," "Little," "Few," or "Low Source of"
An amount that would allow frequent consumption of the food without exceeding the Daily Value for the nutrient, but can only make the claim as it applies to all similar foods

"Good Source Of," "More," or "Added"
The food provides 10% more of the Daily Value for a given nutrient than the comparison food

HELPFUL HINTS AND TIPS

1 Stay challenged when working out alone. Record your best time when walking, running, biking, or swimming, then aim to beat it with the next workout.

2 Make sure you breathe correctly as you exercise. Holding your breath will raise your blood pressure and leave you feeling lightheaded.

3 Mix up your workout to give your muscles a challenge. It will also help overcome boredom.

4 Get in the habit of drinking water before, during, and after your workout.

5 Jack La Lanne's life lessons: *Do something healthy and positive each day.* "Whether you take a long walk at lunch or opt for the stairs instead of the elevator, little things do make a difference." *Concentrate on the moment.* "Don't worry if you missed a day of exercise yesterday. Put all your energy into what you're doing today and what you'll do tomorrow. *Be a role model.* "Motivate your friends and loved ones to stick to their routines by being supportive. You can become their workout partner or listen to and be proud of what they've accomplished."

6 People who carry extra pounds in the abdomen are at greater risk for heart disease, diabetes, and stroke.

7 Working out throughout the day helps to keep your metabolism more active, which burns more calories.

8 Make sure to get at least seven to eight hours of good sleep a night. Studies show that if you are lacking sleep your body will produce less Leptin (a hormone that makes you feel full).

9 Caffeine stays in your system for seven hours. Keep it to a minimum if sleep is a problem.

10 For sustained energy levels, eat five or six small healthy meals a day.

11 Take a stash of healthy snacks when you are on the go.

12 If you know you will be working late, take your dinner along with your lunch and snacks in a small cooler.

13 Adults need at least 130 grams of carbs daily. Sorry, Mr. Atkins.

14 Small amounts of trans fats may elevate heart-disease risk. There is no safe limit known.

15 A 145-pound woman needs to take in 1,423 calories a day just to stay alive.

16 Visualize success in order to become successful.

17 Don't be afraid to work out at work. Hit the floor for a set of push-ups during a break.

18 It is not possible to get a sufficient amount of vitamins E and C from your diet alone. You need to supplement with a good food-based multivitamin.

19 Avoid buffets! Going to one only encourages overeating.

20 Brush your teeth after every meal. When your mouth feels clean, you won't feel like indulging in food any longer.

21 Perform Transformetrics in front of a mirror to receive maximum results. The contractions will be easier to achieve once you see how the muscles work.

22 According to a study at the Cooper Institute for Aerobics Research in Dallas, Texas, it has been estimated that about 150,000 people a year die as a result of inactivity. A sedentary lifestyle is almost as serious a health risk as smoking cigarettes or driving after drinking alcohol.

23 Believe it or not, exercise decreases appetite.

24 Keep in mind: "What you eat today will be walking and talking tomorrow."

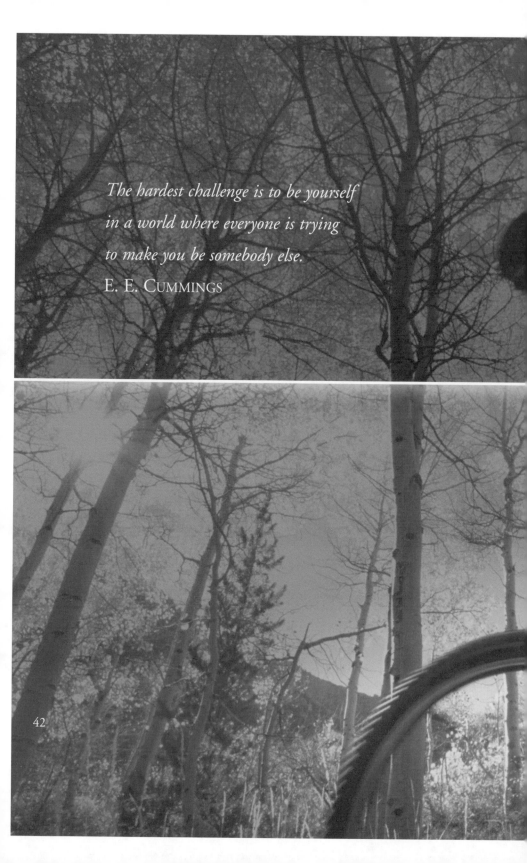

*The hardest challenge is to be yourself
in a world where everyone is trying
to make you be somebody else.*
E. E. CUMMINGS

42

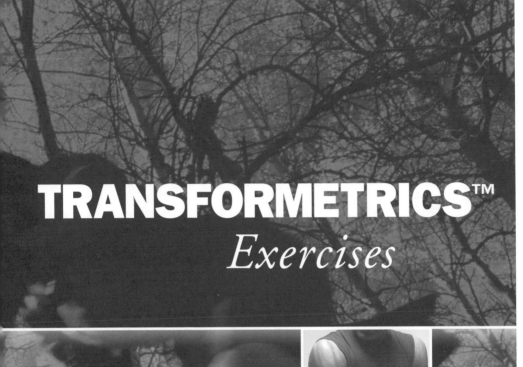

TRANSFORMETRICS™
Exercises

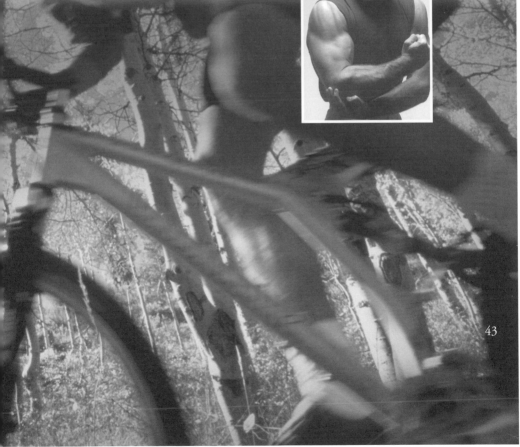

43

TRANSFORMETRICS™ EXERCISES

I f you are living a sedentary lifestyle, you need to hear this. You were not designed by God to sit at a desk for 8+ hours a day and then plop down in front of the television for the evening. Any body that is bound in inactivity while calories are being poured in is headed for trouble. You need to get up and start burning some extra calories.

For instance, a 140-pound woman who is doing light work around the house will burn 240 calories an hour in contrast to 80 calories per hour while sitting. If she is on a brisk walk, she'll burn 370 calories per hour. Up that to 580 calories per hour if she's jogging (a 9-minute mile). A man will burn slightly more calories than a woman while doing the same activity. The point is that calories taken in must be burned or they'll be turned to fat.

There are countless ways to begin exercising. There's walking, jogging, cycling, swimming, calisthenics, dance, hiking, skating, tennis, basketball, aerobics, martial arts, and on and on. We recommend you consider 30 minutes of walking a day for instant calorie burning, plus our Transformetrics™ exercises for strength building to convert fat into muscle and keep your metabolism primed. Both bring tremendous health benefits and are very doable exercises that cost you nothing.

You need to realize that as we age it's easy to gain fat if you don't exercise correctly. Studies tell us that between the ages of 20 and 30, without weight-resistant exercise, we begin to lose muscle. As we age, the rate of muscle loss seems to increase slightly. And as we lose muscle, our basal metabolic rate slows down, which means we burn fewer calories and gain fat. For instance, let's say that between the ages of 30 and 40, we have lost 10 pounds of muscle and replaced it with about 10 pounds of fat. That means that in 10 years, we would have a 20-pound body composition change and still weigh the same amount. But we've changed two dress sizes or added another pant's size.

Strength-building exercise is the only way to reverse this effect of aging. The average person should train their musculature system at least three to four times a week to help maintain a lean body mass and to reap the abundance of health benefits that accompany it—decreasing the risk of osteoporosis, developing and maintaining coordination and balance, and preventing injuries resulting from weak muscles.

There is another interesting aspect to muscle. Did you know that one pound of muscle burns 35 calories a day, whereas one pound of fat burns a paltry 2 calories? Just think, by increasing your muscle or your lean body mass by 10 pounds, you would increase your metabolic rate by about 350 calories a day. Just gaining 5 pounds of muscle would increase your calorie expenditure by 175 calories a day—naturally. That's 63,875 calories or 18 pounds a year! And muscle is denser and takes up much less space than fat. You could therefore maintain the same weight you are now and be 2 sizes smaller by gaining 10 pounds of muscle and losing 10 pounds of fat!

Aerobic Exercise

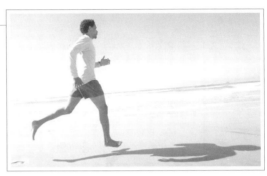

Check with your doctor regarding any form of exercise program you intend to begin. If you are over 40 and in poor health, a treadmill test is highly recommended. A physician or exercise specialist can provide this test that checks blood pressure and uses an electrocardiogram to monitor heart performance. If you ever have symptoms such as chest pain or pressure, heart irregularity, or unusual shortness of breath, call your doctor immediately.

Aerobic exercise, such as walking, is any activity requiring oxygen that uses large muscle groups, is rhythmic in nature, and can be maintained for a period of time. Done consistently, aerobic activity trains the heart, lungs, and cardiovascular system to process and deliver oxygen in a more efficient manner. Whether your goal is weight loss or general health, the longer the duration of your exercise, the more calories you burn.

Start out slowly. If you are really out of shape, it will take time to restore your health. Begin your physical activity program with short sessions (5 to 10 minutes) of physical activity and gradually build up to the desired level of activity (30 minutes). Don't overdo it. Pushing too hard can lead to damage. The same moderate amount of activity can be obtained in longer sessions of moderately intense activities (such as 30 minutes of brisk walking) as in shorter sessions of more strenuous activities (such as 15 to 20 minutes of jogging). You just need to be consistent.

Most experts agree that 3 to 5 aerobic sessions per week for a duration of at least 20 minutes at 60 to 85 percent of your age-specific maximum heart rate is a good place to start. Beginning exercisers would start lower in their target zone. Aim for a heart rate between 70 and 80 percent of the maximum for your age group. If you need to lose weight, you can achieve the greatest loss if you aim for about 60 percent of your maximum heart rate and exercise for 45 to 60 minutes 3 to 5 times a week.

Age	70–80% of Max Rate	60% of Max Rate
20	140–160	120
30	133–152	114
40	126–144	108
50	119–136	102
60	112–128	96
70	105–120	90

Drink water—before, during, and after exercise, especially during warm weather. Replacing water lost by sweating is crucial.

Always warm up for 3 to 5 minutes before stretching. Then stretch out for 3 or 4 minutes before exercising. Stretching the Achilles tendons and the hamstrings should always be included in a warmup. Properly stretching your muscles lessens the likelihood of any muscles being damaged and increases your flexibility. If you are over 60, it's good to walk for about one-quarter mile before stretching.

Cool down for five minutes after working out. Just keep walking around slowly. Don't lie down or sit. And never go directly into a sauna or steam room after exercising. The heat increase can cause heart problems right after exercise.

Transformetrics™ Exercises

Walking is great for burning calories but not for building or replacing muscle. By following the exercises of Transformetrics™ Training System outlined here, Wendie and I will show you how to begin to achieve the strength, fitness, and vitality you've always dreamed of having. And you can do it without having to join a gym, buy expensive equipment, or waste a moment doing anything that doesn't deliver a maximum return on your investment of time. Best of all, you won't be doing anything that will compromise your body, cause pain or injury, create overuse symptoms, or leave you feeling drained rather than energized.

Super Joint and Lifelong Pain-Free Mobility Exercises

As you know from reading the previous pages, the proper nutrition goes hand in hand with using the Transformetrics™ Training System. It is also extremely important to provide mobility and lubrication to all the major joints of the body to obtain optimal strength.

We have included sixteen warm-up exercises that will allow you to achieve mobility in the joints as well provide an incredible stretch of all the major muscle groups from head to toe. The recommended repetition for each joint mobility exercise is at least seven. This allows you to listen to your body and give immediate attention to areas that may have pain from recent or past injuries.

These exercises should be practiced many times throughout the day, every day, to achieve lifelong pain-free mobility. Wouldn't it be nice to be able to wake up in the morning without that stiff achy feeling? Now you can!

Recently, one of our "forum faithfuls" on www.bronzebowpublishing.com commented on how joint mobility movements alone have brought a newfound strength and energy to his life. Matter of fact, many chiropractors and orthopedic surgeons are members on our forum, and they promote joint mobility exercises on a regular basis to their clients. Saying that, need we say more?

We highly recommend that you purchase our book, *The Miracle Seven*, as the next step in your exercise advancement. It utilizes time-tested body sculpting techniques along with high-tension Isometrics that literally allow you to become your own gym.

Let's get to the exercises that you can do anytime and anywhere!

#1 Three Plan Neck Movement

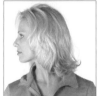 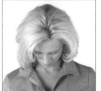

Look right   Look left   Forward   Backward

Side to side

#2 Neck Circles

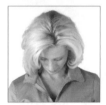 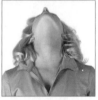

7 slow circles in each direction.

#3 Shoulder Rolls

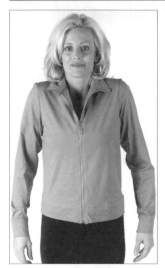 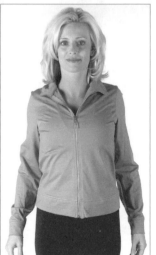 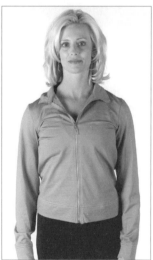

Raise shoulders up (toward ears), back, and around.
7 slow reps. Then up, forward, and around.

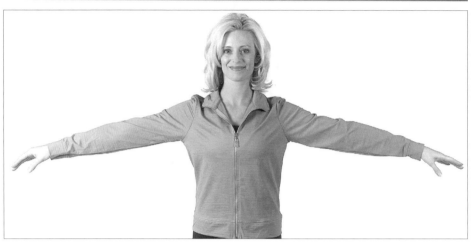

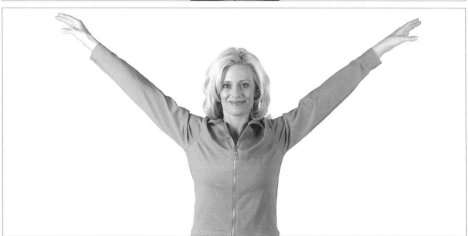

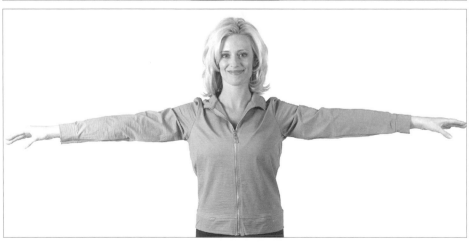

7 reps up, back, and around, then 7 reps up, forward, and around.

#5 Elbow Rotation

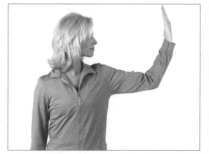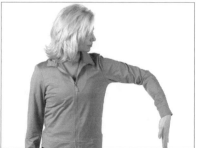

*Begin in "up" position, hand follows a half-circle path down
and half-circle back to up position. 7 reps each arm.*

#6 The Egyptian

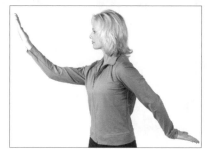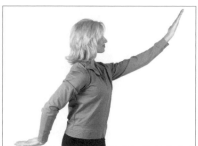

Note: *Both palms face "up" as you twist and pivot from side to side.*

#7 Wrist Rotation

Rotate wrist slowly in both directions. 7 reps each way.

#8 Hands and Fingers

*Stretch and strengthen fingers and wrists by
applying heavy tension and then relaxing.*

#9 Torso Twist

 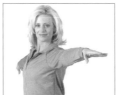 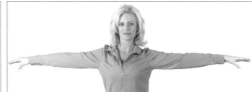

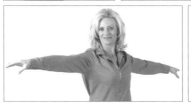 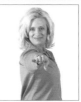

#10 Torso Rotation

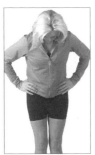 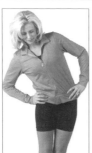 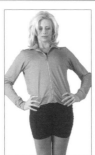 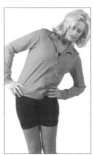 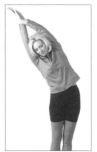

#11 Bend, Stretch, and Touch

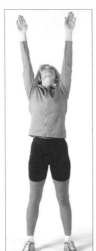 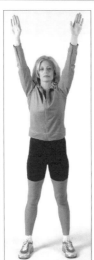 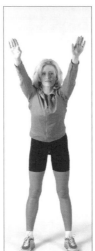 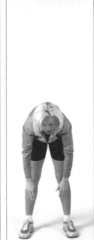 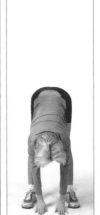

Stand 18" to 24" from a wall. Bend backward and slowly touch the wall behind you, then bend forward and try to touch the floor. Just 7 reps is all that is neccessary.

#12 Hip Rotation

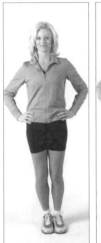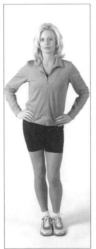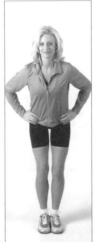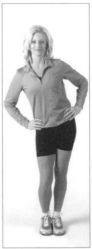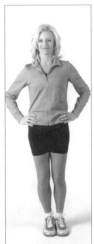

This is a circular motion. 7 reps each direction.

#13 Half Knee Bend

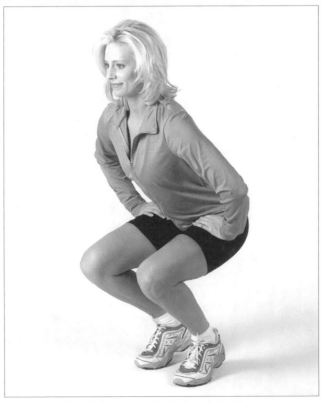

Bend down slowly, but only halfway.

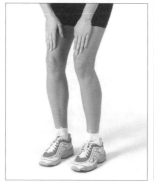 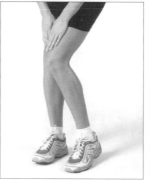 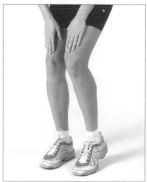

Bend forward and slowly rotate your knees in a circular movement both to the left and right. (Range of motion is limited, so don't push it too far.)

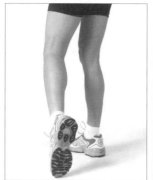 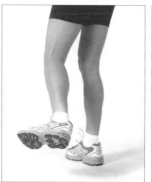 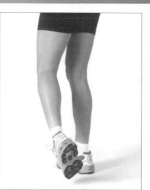

Rotate each ankle in each direction in small semi-circular movement. 7 reps and switch legs.

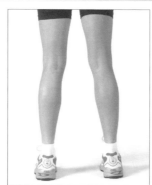 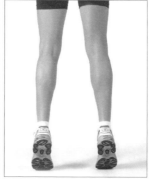

Slowly raise up and down on toes. Just 7 reps is all that is neccessary.

The first step toward success is taken when
you refuse to be a captive of the environment
in which you first find yourself.
MARK CAINE

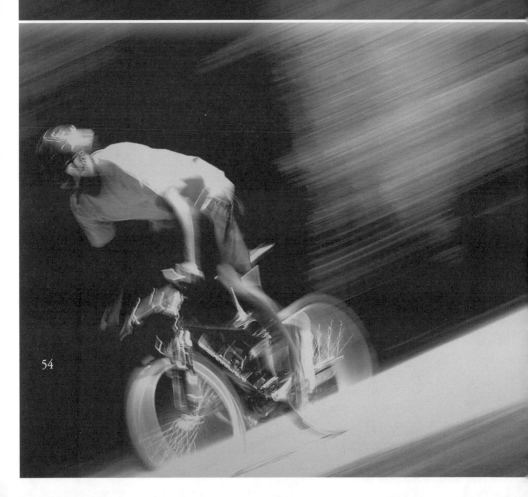

the
60–Day *Journal*

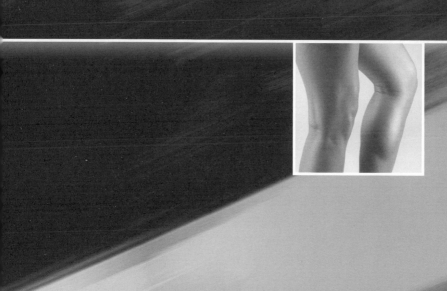

HOW TO USE THE DAILY PLANNER

One of the purposes of the Daily Planner is to provide you with a *simple* format to keep track of the foods you are eating. In contrast to other planners that fix your attention on recording calories, fat grams, carbohydrate grams, protein grams, or saturated fat grams, our goal is for you to bring your eating habits in line with the 80-15-5 Food Plan that was outlined in the Nutritional Transformation chapter. If you review the plan, you'll recall that our goal is for you to make 80 percent of your food choices from Wendie's Lists 1 & 2; 15 percent from List 3; and 5 percent from Lists 4 & 5. If you stay within these simple guidelines, you'll get lean, sculpted, and muscular on the hurry up.

Here's how you make it work. Let's say that for breakfast you had steel cut oatmeal, and two poached eggs over spinach. Write it down in your daily chart. Then go to the Lists and you'll discover you can check off "1 & 2" for the oatmeal, orange juice, and banana and a "3" for the egg. That's a great start to your day, and it's delicious.

Once you get familiar with the Lists, recording these is a breeze. If you eat something that's not on our Lists, you can either use your common sense and compare it to another food on one of the Lists that's like it, or you can go to the back of the Journal and look it up in the Comprehensive Nutritional Chart. This chart lists the calories, total fat, saturated fat, cholesterol, carbohydrates, and cholesterol. From this chart you should be able to classify it within our List numbering system. If it's a fast food, go to the Fast Food Nutritional Chart and check out what's in it. (Chances are you're ringing up a "4 & 5" List item on the fast foods.)

At the end of the day, all you have to do is tally up the number of checks in each column and see how you fared as far as your percentages. For instance, if you have 20 entries for the day, you want 16 of them from Lists 1 & 2; 3 entries from List 3; 1 from Lists 4 & 5. That is aggressive and challenging, we realize, but if you're purposeful in your choices, you'll love the food and you'll especially love the changes it brings to your body.

We've also dedicated a column to "Calories" for anyone who wants to be more exacting. It's also a good safeguard to make certain that you are not cutting back in your eating so much that you are not giving your body the calories it needs to function. If you are eating the right foods but not enough calories, your body will actually begin to consume muscle along with fat in order to compensate. While it varies from person to person, most people need about 12 to 15 calories per pound of body weight per day to maintain their current weight. Obviously, if your goal is a reduction in weight, you'll need to reduce the calories.

A caloric intake below 1,500 calories for men and 1,200 for women is not recommended as diets these low are usually nutritionally deficient. Most men can lose 1 to 2 pounds a week on 1,700 to 2,000 calories a day. Most women can lose 1 to 2 pounds a week on 1,200 to 1,500 calories.

We also want you to record the exercise you did on any given day. You'll find it's a great incentive to get into a regular routine, burn the calories and fat, and build muscle.

What we really hope you'll do, though, is evaluate your day and list "Your Thoughts" in a reflective manner. What did you feel like as you made right choices…and wrong choices? How did you feel after you exercised? What would you do different if you could redo your day? What are you discovering about yourself in this process? What lessons are you going to apply tomorrow? Our intent here is for you to make this journal your own, to put your signature on it, and to reshape your life for the good.

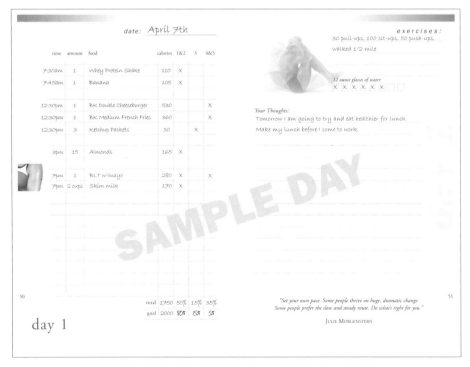

date: April 7th

exercises:
30 pull-ups, 100 sit-ups, 50 push-ups,
walked 1/2 mile

time	amount	food	calories	1&2	3	4&5
7:30am	1	Whey Protein Shake	110	X		
7:45am	1	Banana	105	X		
12:30pm	1	B.K. Double Cheeseburger	530			X
12:30pm	1	B.K. Medium French Fries	360			X
12:30pm	3	Ketchup Packets	30		X	
3pm	15	Almonds	165	X		
7pm	1	BLT w/mayo	280	X		X
7pm	2 cups	Skim milk	170	X		

12 ounce glasses of water:
X X X X X

Your Thoughts:
Tomorrow I am going to try and eat healthier for lunch.
Make my lunch before I come to work.

SAMPLE DAY

				total	1750	50%	15%	35%
				goal	2000	80%	15%	5%

"Set your own pace. Some people thrive on huge, dramatic change.
Some people prefer the slow and steady route. Do what's right for you."

JULIE MORGENSTERN

50

51

day 1

date: _____

time	amount	food	calories	1&2	3	4&5
total						
goal				80%	15%	5%

day 1

12 ounce glasses of water:

☐ ☐ ☐ ☐ ☐ ☐ ☐ ☐

Your Thoughts:

*"Set your own pace. Some people thrive on huge, dramatic change.
Some people prefer the slow and steady route. Do what's right for you."*

JULIE MORGENSTERN

date: _____

time	amount	food	calories	1&2	3	4&5
total						
goal				80%	15%	5%

day 2

_____

_____

_____

_____

12 ounce glasses of water:

☐ ☐ ☐ ☐ ☐ ☐ ☐ ☐

day

Your Thoughts:

_____

_____

_____

_____

_____

_____

_____

_____

_____

_____

_____

_____

_____

_____

_____

"We have one life to live—
and one chance to live it
in the richest way possible."

JUDITH THURMAN

61

date: _____

time	amount	food	calories	1&2	3	4&5
total						
goal				80%	15%	5%

day 3

12 ounce glasses of water:

☐ ☐ ☐ ☐ ☐ ☐ ☐ ☐

Your Thoughts:

"Release the need to blame anyone, including yourself.
We're all doing the best we can with the understanding,
knowledge, and awareness we have."

LOUISE L. HAY

time	amount	food	calories	1&2	3	4&5
			total			
			goal	80%	15%	5%

day 4

12 ounce glasses of water:

☐ ☐ ☐ ☐ ☐ ☐ ☐ ☐ ☐ ☐

Your Thoughts:

*"We're all here for a purpose. Meditate on your mission,
then use your gifts and talents to live your life on purpose.
In doing so, you'll become an unending magnet for miracles."*

TAVIS SMILEY

time	amount	food	calories	1&2	3	4&5
		total				
		goal		80%	15%	5%

day 5

12 ounce glasses of water:

day 05

Your Thoughts:

"Look for things to feel good about, and watch how everything in your life will unfold to reflect that good-feeling vibration."

ABRAHAM-HICKS

time	amount	food	calories	1&2	3	4&5
total						
goal				80%	15%	5%

day 6

12 ounce glasses of water:
☐ ☐ ☐ ☐ ☐ ☐ ☐ ☐ ☐

Your Thoughts:

"It's easy to get lost in endless speculation. So today, release the need to know
why things happen as they do. Instead, ask for the insight
to recognize what you're meant to learn."

CAROLYN MYSS AND PETER OCCHIOGROSSO

time	amount	food	calories	1&2	3	4&5
			total			
			goal	80%	15%	5%

day 7

12 ounce glasses of water:

Your Thoughts:

*"The key to happiness is realizing that it's not what happens
to you that matters, it's how you choose to respond."*

KEITH D. HARRELL

time	amount	food	calories	1&2	3	4&5
total						
goal				80%	15%	5%

day 8

12 ounce glasses of water:

☐ ☐ ☐ ☐ ☐ ☐ ☐ ☐

day 08

Your Thoughts:

*"Always know when you've pushed beyond your limits,
and then bring yourself back to balance."*

LEON NACSON

date: _____

time	amount	food	calories	1&2	3	4&5
		total				
		goal		80%	15%	5%

day 9

12 ounce glasses of water:

Your Thoughts:

*"Set a goal, write it down, and release the outcome.
Small steps make a big difference."*

CHERYL RICHARDSON

date: _____

time	amount	food	calories	1&2	3	4&5
total						
goal				80%	15%	5%

day 10

12 ounce glasses of water:

☐ ☐ ☐ ☐ ☐ ☐ ☐ ☐

Your Thoughts:

"You're more powerful than you realize.
It's safe for you to be powerful!"

DOREEN VIRTUE, PH.D.

time	amount	food	calories	1&2	3	4&5
		total				
		goal		80%	15%	5%

day 11

12 ounce glasses of water:

☐ ☐ ☐ ☐ ☐ ☐ ☐ ☐

day

Your Thoughts:

*"People are constantly changing and growing.
Don't cling to a limited, disconnected, negative image
of a person in the past. See that person now."*

BRIAN L. WEISS, M.D.

time	amount	food	calories	1&2	3	4&5
			total			
			goal	80%	15%	5%

day 12

_____

_____

_____

_____

_____

12 ounce glasses of water:
☐ ☐ ☐ ☐ ☐ ☐ ☐ ☐

Your Thoughts:

_____

_____

_____

_____

_____

_____

_____

_____

_____

_____

_____

_____

_____

*"Be confident and modest about your own merits,
and understand your limitations."*

CHERIE CARTER-SCOTT, PH.D.

time	amount	food	calories	1&2	3	4&5
			total			
			goal	80%	15%	5%

day 13

12 ounce glasses of water:

☐ ☐ ☐ ☐ ☐ ☐ ☐ ☐

Your Thoughts:

83

*"God cannot give us happiness and peace apart from himself,
because it is not there. There is no such thing."*

C. S. LEWIS

date:_____

time	amount	food	calories	1&2	3	4&5
total						
goal				80%	15%	5%

day 14

12 ounce glasses of water:

day 14

Your Thoughts:

"Know that you are the perfect age. Each year is special and precious, for you shall only live it once. Be comfortable with growing older."

LOUISE L. HAY

time	amount	food	calories	1&2	3	4&5
total						
goal				80%	15%	5%

day 15

12 ounce glasses of water:

☐ ☐ ☐ ☐ ☐ ☐ ☐ ☐

Your Thoughts:

"If you don't move your body, your brain thinks you're dead.
Movement of the body will not only clear out the sludge,
but will also give you more energy. Treat your body like a car—
keep it tuned up and it will run for a very long time."

SYLVIA BROWNE

date: _____

time	amount	food	calories	1&2	3	4&5
			total			
			goal	80%	15%	5%

day 16

_____

_____

_____

_____

12 ounce glasses of water: ☑ ☐ ☐ ☑ ☐ ☐ ☐ ☐

Your Thoughts:

_____

_____

_____

_____

_____

_____

_____

_____

_____

_____

_____

_____

"*Do not pray for easy lives. Pray to be stronger men.
Do not pray for tasks equal to your powers. Pray for powers equal to your tasks.*"
PHILLIPS BROOKS

*date:*_____

time	amount	food	calories	1&2	3	4&5
total						
goal				80%	15%	5%

day 17

12 ounce glasses of water:

☐ ☐ ☐ ☐ ☐ ☐ ☐ ☐

day

17

Your Thoughts:

91

*"Care for your body. Self-love and self-acceptance
are the ultimate acts of self-care."*

CHERYL RICHARDSON

date:_____

time	amount	food	calories	1&2	3	4&5
total						
goal				80%	15%	5%

day 18

12 ounce glasses of water:

☐ ☐ ☐ ☐ ☐ ☐ ☐ ☐

Your Thoughts:

*"When you accept the fact that the only constant is change,
you'll no longer be willing to do damage to yourself and others
by refusing to accept it. Welcoming change is welcoming life."*

ANNE WILSON SCHAEF

*date:*_____

time	amount	food	calories	1&2	3	4&5
			total			
			goal	80%	15%	5%

day 19

12 ounce glasses of water:

☐ ☐ ☐ ☐ ☐ ☐ ☐ ☐

Your Thoughts:

_"Treat your body with respect by feeding it nourishing and nutritious foods.
If you're good to your body, it will be good to you."_

SYLVIA BROWNE

time	amount	food	calories	1&2	3	4&5
		total				
		goal		80%	15%	5%

day 20

exercises:

12 ounce glasses of water:

day 20

Your Thoughts:

97

"Success is never ending, failure is never final."
DR. ROBERT SCHULLER

time	amount	food	calories	1&2	3	4&5
total						
goal				80%	15%	5%

day 21

12 ounce glasses of water:

☐ ☐ ☐ ☐ ☐ ☐ ☐ ☐

Your Thoughts:

*"In my opinion, a woman doesn't deserve the title of 'supermodel'
until she proves she can actually fly."*

THE COVERT COMIC

date: _____

time	amount	food	calories	1&2	3	4&5
total						
goal				80%	15%	5%

day 22

12 ounce glasses of water:
☐ ☐ ☐ ☐ ☐ ☐ ☐ ☐

Your Thoughts:

101

"You can't control the wind, but you can adjust your sails."

AUTHOR UNKNOWN

time	amount	food	calories	1&2	3	4&5
		total				
		goal		80%	15%	5%

day 23

12 ounce glasses of water:

☐ ☐ ☐ ☐ ☐ ☐ ☐ ☐

day 23

Your Thoughts:

103

"Even if you're on the right track, you'll get run over if you just sit there."

WILL ROGERS

date:_____

time	amount	food	calories	1&2	3	4&5
total						
goal				80%	15%	5%

day 24

12 ounce glasses of water:

☐ ☐ ☐ ☐ ☐ ☐ ☐ ☐

Your Thoughts:

"The first wealth is health."

RALPH WALDO EMERSON

time	amount	food	calories	1&2	3	4&5
			total			
			goal	80%	15%	5%

day 25

12 ounce glasses of water:

☐ ☐ ☐ ☐ ☐ ☐ ☐ ☐

Your Thoughts:

"To wish to be well is a part of becoming well."

ALEXANDER POPE

time	amount	food	calories	1&2	3	4&5
		total				
		goal		80%	15%	5%

day 26

12 ounce glasses of water:

☐ ☐ ☐ ☐ ☐ ☐ ☐ ☐

day 26

Your Thoughts:

109

"To get rich never risk your health.
For it is the truth that health is the wealth of wealth."

GREG ANDERSON

time	amount	food	calories	1&2	3	4&5
total						
goal				80%	15%	5%

day 27

12 ounce glasses of water:

☐ ☐ ☐ ☐ ☐ ☐ ☐ ☐

Your Thoughts:

111

*"The healthy, strong individual is the one who asks for help when he needs it.
Whether he has an abscess on his knee or in his soul."*

RICHARD BAKER

date: _____

time	amount	food	calories	1&2	3	4&5
total						
goal				80%	15%	5%

day 28

12 ounce glasses of water:

☐ ☐ ☐ ☐ ☐ ☐ ☐ ☐

Your Thoughts:

"Nothing great was ever achieved without enthusiasm."

RALPH WALDO EMERSON

date: _____

time	amount	food	calories	1&2	3	4&5
	total					
	goal			80%	15%	5%

day 29

12 ounce glasses of water:

☐ ☐ ☐ ☐ ☐ ☐ ☐ ☐

day 29

Your Thoughts:

"Our mental and emotional diets determine our overall energy levels, health, and well-being more than we realize. Every thought and feeling, no matter how big or small, impacts our inner energy reserves."

DOC CHILDRE

time	amount	food	calories	1&2	3	4&5
total						
goal				80%	15%	5%

day 30

12 ounce glasses of water:

☐ ☐ ☐ ☐ ☐ ☐ ☐ ☐

Your Thoughts:

*"There is more hunger for love and appreciation
in this world than for bread."*

MOTHER TERESA

date:

time	amount	food	calories	1&2	3	4&5
total						
goal				80%	15%	5%

day 31

12 ounce glasses of water:

☐ ☐ ☐ ☐ ☐ ☐ ☐ ☐

Your Thoughts:

*"A harmonious relationship with one you love can enhance
your work, health, and entire well-being."*

DOC CHILDRE

time	amount	food	calories	1&2	3	4&5
		total				
		goal		80%	15%	5%

day 32

12 ounce glasses of water:

☐ ☐ ☐ ☐ ☐ ☐ ☐ ☐

day 32

Your Thoughts:

121

"A sad soul can kill you quicker than a germ."

JOHN STEINBECK

time	amount	food	calories	1&2	3	4&5
total						
goal				80%	15%	5%

day 33

12 ounce glasses of water:

☐ ☐ ☐ ☐ ☐ ☐ ☐ ☐ ☐

Your Thoughts:

"_Love cures people—both the ones who give it and the ones who receive it._"

DR. KARL MENNINGER

time	amount	food	calories	1&2	3	4&5
			total			
			goal	80%	15%	5%

day 34

12 ounce glasses of water:

Your Thoughts:

"He who has health has hope; and he who has hope has everything."

ARABIAN PROVERB

time	amount	food	calories	1&2	3	4&5
total						
goal				80%	15%	5%

day 35

12 ounce glasses of water:

☐ ☐ ☐ ☐ ☐ ☐ ☐ ☐

day 35

Your Thoughts:

127

"Health is the thing that makes you feel that now is the best time of the year."

FRANKLIN ADAMS

date: _____

time	amount	food	calories	1&2	3	4&5
total						
goal				80%	15%	5%

day 36

12 ounce glasses of water:

Your Thoughts:

"The person who sends out positive thoughts activates the world around him positively and draws back to himself positive results."

NORMAN VINCENT PEALE

time	amount	food	calories	1&2	3	4&5
total						
goal				80%	15%	5%

day 37

_____

_____

_____

_____

12 ounce glasses of water:
☐ ☐ ☐ ☐ ☐ ☐ ☐ ☐

Your Thoughts:

_____

_____

_____

_____

_____

_____

_____

_____

_____

_____

_____

_____

_____

> *"If you focus on results, you will never change.*
> *If you focus on change, you will get results."*
>
> JACK DIXON

date: _____

time	amount	food	calories	1&2	3	4&5
		total				
		goal		80%	15%	5%

day 38

12 ounce glasses of water:

☐ ☐ ☐ ☐ ☐ ☐ ☐ ☐

day 38

Your Thoughts:

133

"Waiting is a trap. There will always be reasons to wait.
The truth is, there are only two things in life, reasons and results,
and reasons simply don't count."

DR. ROBERT ANTHONY

date:

time	amount	food	calories	1&2	3	4&5
		total				
		goal		80%	15%	5%

day 39

12 ounce glasses of water:

☐ ☐ ☐ ☐ ☐ ☐ ☐ ☐

Your Thoughts:

*"It is inevitable that some defeat will enter even the most victorious life.
The human spirit is never finished when it is defeated....
It is finished when it surrenders."*

BEN STEIN

date: _____

time	amount	food	calories	1&2	3	4&5
total						
goal				80%	15%	5%

day 40

12 ounce glasses of water:
□ □ □ □ □ □ □ □

Your Thoughts:

"How many a man has thrown up his hands at a time when a little more effort, a little more patience would have achieved success?"

ELBERT HUBBARD

*date:*_____

time	amount	food	calories	1&2	3	4&5
total						
goal				80%	15%	5%

day 41

12 ounce glasses of water:

☐ ☐ ☐ ☐ ☐ ☐ ☐ ☐ ☐

day 41

Your Thoughts:

*"I do not think that there is any other quality so essential
to success of any kind as the quality of perseverance.
It overcomes almost everything, even nature."*

JOHN D. ROCKEFELLER

time	amount	food	calories	1&2	3	4&5
total						
goal				80%	15%	5%

day 42

12 ounce glasses of water:

☐ ☐ ☐ ☐ ☐ ☐ ☐ ☐

Your Thoughts:

141

"Obstacles can't stop you. Problems can't stop you.
Most of all other people can't stop you. Only you can stop you."

JEFFREY GITOMER

time	amount	food	calories	1&2	3	4&5
		total				
		goal		80%	15%	5%

day 43

12 ounce glasses of water:

☐ ☐ ☐ ☐ ☐ ☐ ☐ ☐

Your Thoughts:

"You become a champion by fighting one more round.
When things are tough, you fight one more round."

JAMES J. CORBETT

date: _____

time	amount	food	calories	1&2	3	4&5
	total					
	goal			80%	15%	5%

day 44

12 ounce glasses of water:

day
44

Your Thoughts:

145

"*The greatest amount of wasted time is the time not getting started.*"

DAWSON TROTMAN

date: _____

time	amount	food	calories	1&2	3	4&5
total						
goal				80%	15%	5%

day 45

12 ounce glasses of water:

☐ ☐ ☐ ☐ ☐ ☐ ☐ ☐

Your Thoughts:

"Everyone has a success mechanism and a failure mechanism. The failure mechanism goes off by itself. The success mechanism only goes off with a goal. Every time we write down and talk about a goal we push the button to start the success mechanism."

CHARLES "TREMENDOUS" JONES

date: _____

time	amount	food	calories	1&2	3	4&5
total						
goal				80%	15%	5%

day 46

12 ounce glasses of water:

☐ ☐ ☐ ☐ ☐ ☐ ☐ ☐

Your Thoughts:

149

"The vision must be followed by the venture.
It is not enough to stare up the steps—we must step up the stairs."

VANCE HAVNER

date:

time	amount	food	calories	1&2	3	4&5
			total			
			goal	80%	15%	5%

150

day 47

exercises:

12 ounce glasses of water:
☐ ☐ ☐ ☐ ☐ ☐ ☐ ☐ ☐

day 47

Your Thoughts:

151

"We cannot do everything at once, but we can do something at once."
CALVIN COOLIDGE

*date:*_____

time	amount	food	calories	1&2	3	4&5
		total				
		goal		80%	15%	5%

day 48

12 ounce glasses of water:

☐ ☐ ☐ ☐ ☐ ☐ ☐ ☐

Your Thoughts:

153

"Know your goal, make a plan, and pull the trigger."

PHIL C. McGRAW

time	amount	food	calories	1&2	3	4&5
total						
goal				80%	15%	5%

154

day 49

12 ounce glasses of water:

☐ ☐ ☐ ☐ ☐ ☐ ☐ ☐

Your Thoughts:

155

"If you want to be happy, set a goal that commands your thoughts,
liberates your energy, and inspires your hopes."

ANDREW CARNEGIE

date: _____

time	amount	food	calories	1&2	3	4&5
total						
goal				80%	15%	5%

day 50

exercises:

12 ounce glasses of water:

day 50

Your Thoughts:

"Crystallize your goals. Make a plan for achieving them and set yourself a deadline. Then, with supreme confidence, determination, and disregard for obstacles and other people's criticisms, carry out your plan."

PAUL MEYER

time	amount	food	calories	1&2	3	4&5
total						
goal				80%	15%	5%

day 51

12 ounce glasses of water:

☐ ☐ ☐ ☐ ☐ ☐ ☐ ☐

Your Thoughts:

"Think little goals and expect little achievements.
Think big goals and win big success."

DAVID J. SCHWARTZ

date: _____

time	amount	food	calories	1&2	3	4&5
total						
goal				80%	15%	5%

day 52

12 ounce glasses of water:
☐ ☐ ☐ ☐ ☐ ☐ ☐ ☐

Your Thoughts:

"Write it down. Written goals have a way of transforming wishes into wants;
can'ts into cans; dreams into plans; and plans into reality.
Don't just think it—ink it!"

AUTHOR UNKNOWN

time	amount	food	calories	1&2	3	4&5
total						
goal				80%	15%	5%

day 53

12 ounce glasses of water:

☐ ☐ ☐ ☐ ☐ ☐ ☐ ☐ ☐

day 53

Your Thoughts:

"It is not how much we have, but how much we enjoy, that makes happiness."

CHARLES SPURGEON

time	amount	food	calories	1&2	3	4&5
			total			
			goal	80%	15%	5%

day 54

12 ounce glasses of water:

☐ ☐ ☐ ☐ ☐ ☐ ☐ ☐

Your Thoughts:

165

"Happiness is inward and not outward; and so it does not depend on what we have, but on what we are."

HENRY VAN DYKE

time	amount	food	calories	1&2	3	4&5
total						
goal				80%	15%	5%

day 55

12 ounce glasses of water:

☐ ☐ ☐ ☐ ☐ ☐ ☐ ☐

Your Thoughts:

167

"Hope sees the invisible, feels the intangible, and achieves the impossible."

AUTHOR UNKNOWN

time	amount	food	calories	1&2	3	4&5
	total					
	goal			80%	15%	5%

day 56

12 ounce glasses of water:

day 56

Your Thoughts:

"Don't go through life, grow through life."

ERIC BUTTERWORTH

time	amount	food	calories	1&2	3	4&5
			total			
			goal	80%	15%	5%

day 57

12 ounce glasses of water:

☐ ☐ ☐ ☐ ☐ ☐ ☐ ☐

Your Thoughts:

171

"The greatest inspiration is often born of desperation."

COMER COTRELL

time	amount	food	calories	1&2	3	4&5
total						
goal				80%	15%	5%

172

day 58

12 ounce glasses of water:

Your Thoughts:

173

day 89

"*The only thing wrong with doing nothing is that
you never know when you're finished.*"

AUTHOR UNKNOWN

time	amount	food	calories	1&2	3	4&5
			total			
			goal	80%	15%	5%

day 59

12 ounce glasses of water:

☐ ☐ ☐ ☐ ☐ ☐ ☐ ☐

day 59

Your Thoughts:

175

"Tomorrow is the only day in the year that appeals to a lazy man."

JIMMY LYONS

time	amount	food	calories	1&2	3	4&5
total						
goal				80%	15%	5%

day 60

12 ounce glasses of water:

☐ ☐ ☐ ☐ ☐ ☐ ☐ ☐

Your Thoughts:

day 60

"Laziness is nothing more than the habit of resting before you get tired."

MORTIMER CAPLAN

Motivation is a fire from within.
If someone else tries to light that fire under you,
chances are it will burn very briefly.

STEPHEN R. COVEY

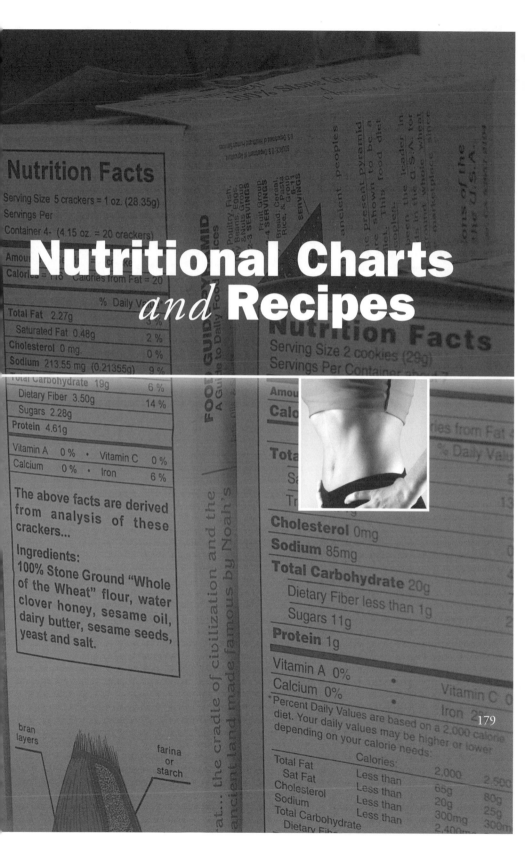

Nutritional Charts *and* Recipes

Nutrition Facts

Serving Size 5 crackers = 1 oz. (28.35g)
Servings Per
Container 4- (4.15 oz. = 20 crackers)

Amount
Calories = 118   Calories from Fat = 20

	% Daily Value
Total Fat 2.27g	3 %
Saturated Fat 0.48g	2 %
Cholesterol 0 mg.	0 %
Sodium 213.55 mg (0.21355g)	9 %
Total Carbohydrate 19g	6 %
Dietary Fiber 3.50g	14 %
Sugars 2.28g	
Protein 4.61g	

Vitamin A 0 %	•	Vitamin C 0 %	
Calcium 0 %	•	Iron 6 %	

The above facts are derived from analysis of these crackers...

Ingredients:
100% Stone Ground "Whole of the Wheat" flour, water clover honey, sesame oil, dairy butter, sesame seeds, yeast and salt.

bran layers

farina or starch

FOOD GUIDE PYRAMID
A Guide to Daily Food Choices

...the cradle of civilization and the ancient land made famous by Noah's

Nutrition Facts

Serving Size 2 cookies (29g)
Servings Per Container about 7

Amount
Calories

Total

Saturated

Trans

Cholesterol 0mg

Sodium 85mg

Total Carbohydrate 20g

Dietary Fiber less than 1g

Sugars 11g

Protein 1g

Vitamin A 0%

Calcium 0%   •   Vitamin C 0

*Percent Daily Values are based on a 2,000 calorie diet. Your daily values may be higher or lower depending on your calorie needs:

		Calories:	2,000	2,500
Total Fat	Less than			
Sat Fat	Less than		65g	80g
Cholesterol	Less than		20g	25g
Sodium	Less than		300mg	300m
Total Carbohydrate			2,400m	
Dietary Fib				

COMPREHENSIVE
NUTRITIONAL CHART

The U.S. Department of Agriculture is the source of all the nutritional information.

Food Item	Amount	Fat Grams	Calories	Carbo Grams	Protein Grams	Chol. Mgs.	Saturated Fat
1000 Island Salad Dressing	1 T	6	60	2	0	4	1
100% Natural cereal	1 oz.	6	135	18	3	0	4.1
40% Bran Flakes, Kellogg's	1 oz.	1	90	22	4	0	.1
40% Bran Flakes, Post	1 oz.	0	90	22	3	0	.1
Alfalfa seeds, sprouted, raw	1 cup	0	10	1	1	0	0
All-Bran cereal	1 oz.	1	70	21	4	0	.1
Almonds, slivered	1 cup	70	795	28	27	0	6.7
Almonds, whole	1 oz.	15	165	6	6	0	1.4
Angel Food Cake, from mix	1 piece	0	125	29	3	0	0
Apple juice, canned	1 cup	0	115	29	0	0	0
Apple pie	1 piece	18	405	60	3	0	4.6
Applesauce, canned, sweetened	1 cup	0	195	51	0	0	.1
Applesauce, canned, unsweetened	1 cup	0	105	28	0	0	0
Apples, raw, peeled, sliced	1 cup	0	65	16	0	0	.1
Apples, raw, unpeeled	1	0	80	21	0	0	.1
Apricots, canned, juice packed	1 cup	0	120	31	2	0	0
Apricots, dried, uncooked	1 cup	1	310	80	5	0	0
Apricots, raw	3	0	50	12	1	0	0
Apricot, canned, heavy syrup	1 cup	0	215	55	1	0	0
Artichokes, globe, cooked	1	0	55	12	3	0	0
Asparagus, cooked from frozen	1 cup	1	50	9	5	0	.2
Asparagus, cooked from raw	1 cup	1	45	8	5	0	.1
Asparagus, canned, spears	4 spears	0	10	2	1	0	0
Avocados, California	1	30	305	12	4	0	4.5
Avocados, Florida	1	27	340	27	5	0	5.3
Bagels, egg	1	2	200	38	7	44	.3
Bagels, plain	1	2	200	38	7	0	.3
Baking powder, low sodium	1 tsp	0	5	1	0	0	0
Baking powder, straight phosphate	1 tsp	0	5	1	0	0	0
Baking powder biscuits, from mix	1	3	95	14	2	0	.8
Baking powder biscuits, home rec.	1	5	100	13	2	0	1.2
Bamboo shoots, canned, drained	1 cup	1	25	4	2	0	.1
Bananas	1	1	105	27	1	0	.2
Bananas, sliced	1 cup	1	140	35	2	0	.3
Barbecue sauce	1 T	0	10	2	0	0	0
Barley, pearled, light, uncooked	1 cup	2	700	158	16	0	.3

Food Item	Amount	Fat Grams	Calories	Carbo Grams	Protein Grams	Chol. Mgs.	Saturated Fat
Bean sprouts, mung, cooked, drain	1 cup	0	25	5	3	0	0
Bean sprouts, mung, raw	1 cup	0	30	6	3	0	0
Bean with bacon soup, canned	1 cup	6	170	23	8	3	1.5
Beans, dry, canned, w/frankfurter	1 cup	18	365	32	19	30	7.4
Beans, dry, can., w/pork+swt. sce.	1 cup	12	385	54	16	10	4.3
Beef and vegetable stew, hm. rec.	1 cup	11	220	15	16	71	4.4
Beef broth, bouillon, cons., canned	1 cup	1	15	0	3	0	.3
Beef gravy, canned	1 cup	5	125	11	9	7	2.7
Beef heart, braised	3 oz.	5	150	0	24	164	1.2
Beef liver, fried	3 oz.	7	185	7	23	410	2.5
Beef noodle soup, canned	1 cup	3	85	9	5	5	1.1
Beef potpie, home recipe	1 piece	30	515	39	21	42	7.9
Beef roast, eye o round, lean	2.6 oz.	5	135	0	22	52	1.9
Beef roast, rib, lean only	2.2 oz.	9	150	0	17	49	3.6
Beef steak, sirloin, broil, lean	2.5 oz.	6	150	0	22	64	2.6
Beef, canned, corned	3 oz.	10	185	0	22	80	4.2
Beef, ckd., bttm. round, lean only	2.8 oz.	8	175	0	25	75	2.7
Beef, ckd., bttm. round, lean+fat	3 oz.	13	220	0	25	81	4.8
Beef, ckd., chuck blade, lean only	2.2 oz.	9	170	0	19	66	3.9
Beef, ckd., chuck blade, lean+fat	3 oz.	26	325	0	22	87	10.8
Beef, dried, chipped	2.5 oz.	4	145	0	24	46	1.8
Beer, light	12 F oz.	0	95	5	1	0	0
Beer, regular	12 F oz.	0	150	13	1	0	0
Beet greens, cooked, drained	1 cup	0	40	8	4	0	0
Beets, canned, drained	1 cup	0	55	12	2	0	0
Beets, cooked, drained, diced	1 cup	0	55	11	2	0	0
Beets, cooked, drained, whole	2 beets	0	30	7	1	0	0
Black beans, dry, cooked, drained	1 cup	1	225	41	15	0	.1
Blackberries, raw	1 cup	1	75	18	1	0	.2
Black-eyed peas, dry, cooked	1 cup	1	190	35	13	0	.2
Black-eyed peas, raw, cooked	1 cup	1	180	30	13	0	.3
Black-eyed peas, frzn., cooked	1 cup	1	225	40	14	0	.3
Blue cheese	1 oz.	8	100	1	6	21	5.3
Blue cheese salad dressing	1 T	8	75	1	1	3	1.5
Blueberries, frozen, sweetened	1 cup	0	185	50	1	0	0
Blueberries, raw	1 cup	1	80	20	1	0	0
Blueberry muffins, home recipe	1	5	135	20	3	19	1.5
Blueberry pie	1 piece	17	380	55	4	0	4.3
Bologna	2 slices	16	180	2	7	31	6.1
Boston brown bread	1 slice	1	95	21	2	3	.3
Bouillon, dehydrated, unprepared	1 pkt	1	15	1	1	1	.3
Bran muffins, home recipe	1	6	125	19	3	24	1.4
Braunschweiger	2 slices	18	205	2	8	89	6.2

Food Item	Amount	Fat Grams	Calories	Carbo Grams	Protein Grams	Chol. Mgs.	Saturated Fat
Brazil nuts	1 oz.	19	185	4	4	0	4.6
Bread stuffing, from mix, dry type	1 cup	31	500	50	9	0	6.1
Bread stuffing, from mix, moist	1 cup	26	420	40	9	67	5.3
Breadcrumbs, dry, grated	1 cup	5	390	73	13	5	1.5
Broccoli, frozen, cooked, drained	1 cup	0	50	10	6	0	0
Broccoli, raw	1 spear	1	40	8	4	0	.1
Broccoli, raw, cooked, drained	1 cup	0	45	9	5	0	.1
Brown and serve sausage	1 link	5	50	0	2	9	1.7
Brown gravy from dry mix	1 cup	2	80	14	3	2	.9
Brownies w/nuts, home recipe	1 sq.	6	95	11	1	18	1.4
Brussels sprouts, frozen, cooked	1 cup	1	65	13	6	0	.1
Brussels sprouts, raw, cooked	1 cup	1	60	13	4	0	.2
Buckwheat flour, light, sifted	1 cup	1	340	78	6	0	.2
Bulgur, uncooked	1 cup	3	600	129	19	0	1.2
Buttermilk, dried	1 cup	7	465	59	41	83	4.3
Buttermilk, fluid	1 cup	2	100	12	8	9	1.3
Butter	1 pat	4	35	0	0	11	2.5
Butter	1 T	11	100	0	0	31	7.1
Cabbage, Chinese, pak-choi, ckd.	1 cup	0	20	3	3	0	0
Cabbage, Chinese, pe-tsai, raw	1 cup	0	10	2	1	0	0
Cabbage, common, cooked	1 cup	0	30	7	1	0	0
Cabbage, common, raw	1 cup	0	15	4	1	0	0
Cabbage, red, raw	1 cup	0	20	4	1	0	0
Cabbage, savoy, raw	1 cup	0	20	4	1	0	0
Cake or pastry flour, sifted	1 cup	1	350	76	7	0	.1
Camembert cheese	1 wedge	9	115	0	8	27	5.8
Cantaloupe, raw	1/2	1	95	22	2	0	.1
Captain Crunch cereal	1 oz.	3	120	23	1	0	1.7
Caramels, plain or chocolate	1 oz.	3	115	22	1	1	2.2
Carob flour	1 cup	0	255	126	6	0	0
Carrot cake, cream cheese frosting	1 piece	21	385	48	4	74	4.1
Carrots, canned	1 cup	0	35	8	1	0	.1
Carrots, cooked, frozen	1 cup	0	55	12	2	0	0
Carrots, cooked, raw	1 cup	0	70	16	2	0	.1
Cashew nuts, dry roasted	1 oz.	13	165	9	4	0	2.6
Cashew nuts, oil roasted	1 oz.	14	165	8	5	0	2.7
Catsup	1 T	0	15	4	0	0	0
Cauliflower, cooked from frozen	1 cup	0	35	7	3	0	.1
Cauliflower, cooked from raw	1 cup	0	30	6	2	0	0
Cauliflower, raw	1 cup	0	25	5	2	0	0
Celery seed	1 tsp	1	10	1	0	0	0
Celery, pascal type, raw, piece	1 cup	0	20	4	1	0	0
Cheddar cheese	1 cu. in.	6	70	0	4	18	3.6

Food Item	Amount	Fat Grams	Calories	Carbo Grams	Protein Grams	Chol. Mgs.	Saturated Fat
Cheddar cheese	1 oz.	9	115	0	7	30	6
Cheddar cheese, shredded	1 cup	37	455	1	28	119	23.8
Cheerios cereal	1 oz.	2	110	20	4	0	.3
Cheese crackers, plain	10	3	50	6	1	6	.9
Cheese sauce w/milk, from mix	1 cup	17	305	23	16	53	9.3
Cheeseburger, 4 oz. patty	1	31	525	40	30	104	15.1
Cheesecake	1 piece	18	280	26	5	170	9.9
Cherries, sour, red, canned, water	1 cup	0	90	22	2	0	.1
Cherries, sweet, raw	10	1	50	11	1	0	.1
Cherry pie	1 piece	18	410	61	4	0	4.7
Chestnuts, European, roasted	1 cup	3	350	76	5	0	.6
Chicken a la king, home recipe	1 cup	34	470	12	27	221	12.9
Chicken and noodles, home recipe	1 cup	18	365	26	22	103	5.1
Chicken chow mein, canned	1 cup	0	95	18	7	8	.1
Chicken chow mein, home recipe	1 cup	10	255	10	31	75	4.1
Chicken frankfurter	1	9	115	3	6	45	2.5
Chicken gravy from dry mix	1 cup	2	85	14	3	3	.5
Chicken gravy, canned	1 cup	14	190	13	5	5	3.4
Chicken liver, cooked	1	1	30	0	5	126	.4
Chicken noodle soup, canned	1 cup	2	75	9	4	7	.7
Chicken noodle soup, dehyd.	1 pkt	1	40	6	2	2	.2
Chicken potpie, home recipe	1 piece	31	545	42	23	56	10.3
Chicken rice soup, canned	1 cup	2	60	7	4	7	.5
Chicken roll, light	2 slices	4	90	1	11	28	1.1
Chicken, canned, boneless	5 oz.	11	235	0	31	88	3.1
Chicken, fried, batter, breast	4.9 oz.	18	365	13	35	119	4.9
Chicken, fried, batter, drumstick	2.5 oz.	11	195	6	16	62	3
Chicken, fried, flour, breast	3.5 oz.	9	220	2	31	87	2.4
Chicken, fried, flour, drumstick	1.7 oz.	7	120	1	13	44	1.8
Chicken, roasted, breast	3 oz.	3	140	0	27	73	.9
Chicken, roasted, drumstick	1.6 oz.	2	75	0	12	41	.7
Chicken, stewed, light + dark	1 cup	9	250	0	38	116	2.6
Chickpeas, cooked, drained	1 cup	4	270	45	15	0	.4
Chili con carne w/beans, canned	1 cup	16	340	31	19	28	5.8
Chili powder	1 tsp	0	10	1	0	0	.1
Chocolate chip cookies	4	11	185	26	2	18	3.9
Chocolate chip cookies, refrig.	4	11	225	32	2	22	4
Chocolate milk, low-fat 1%	1 cup	3	160	26	8	7	1.5
Chocolate milk, low-fat 2%	1 cup	5	180	26	8	17	3.1
Chocolate milk, regular	1 cup	8	210	26	8	31	5.3
Chocolate, bitter	1 oz.	15	145	8	3	0	9
Chip suey w/beef + pork, home rec.	1 cup	17	300	13	26	68	4.3
Cinnamon	1 tsp	0	5	2	0	0	0

Food Item	Amount	Fat Grams	Calories	Carbo Grams	Protein Grams	Chol. Mgs.	Saturated Fat
Clam chowder, Manhattan, canned	1 cup	2	80	12	4	2	.4
Clam chowder, New Eng., w/milk	1 cup	7	165	17	9	22	3
Clams, canned, drained	3 oz.	2	85	2	13	54	.5
Clams, raw	3 oz.	1	65	2	11	43	.3
Club soda	12 F oz.	0	0	0	0	0	0
Cocoa pwdr. w/o no-fat dry milk	1 serv.	9	225	30	9	33	5.4
Cocoa pwdr. w/no-fat dry milk	1 serv.	1	100	22	3	1	.6
Coconut, dried, sweet., shredded	1 cup	33	470	44	3	0	29.3
Coconut, raw, piece	1 piece	15	160	7	1	0	13.4
Coconut, raw, shredded	1 cup	27	285	12	3	0	23.8
Coffee cake, crumb, from mix	1 piece	7	230	38	5	47	2
Coffee, brewed	6 F oz.	0	0	0	0	0	0
Coffee, instant, prepared	6 F oz.	0	0	1	0	0	0
Cola, diet, aspartame only	12 F oz.	0	0	0	0	0	0
Cola, diet, saccharin only	12 F oz.	0	0	0	0	0	0
Cola, regular	12 F oz.	0	160	41	0	0	0
Collards, cooked from frozen	1 cup	1	60	12	5	0	.1
Collards, cooked from raw	1 cup	0	25	5	2	0	.1
Cooked salad dressing, home rec.	1 T	2	25	2	1	9	.5
Corn chips	1 oz.	9	155	16	2	0	1.4
Corn Flakes, Kellogg's	1 oz.	0	110	24	2	0	0
Corn grits, cooked, instant	1 pkt	0	80	18	2	0	0
Corn grits, ckd., yellow or white	1 cup	0	145	31	3	0	0
Corn muffins, home recipe	1	5	145	21	3	23	1.5
Corn oil	1 T	14	125	0	0	0	1.8
Cornmeal, bolted, dry form	1 cup	4	440	91	11	0	.5
Cornmeal, degermed, enriched, ck.	1 cup	0	120	26	3	0	0
Cornmeal, degermed, enriched, dry	1 cup	2	500	108	11	0	.2
Cornmeal, whole-grnd., unbolt, dry	1 cup	5	435	90	11	0	.5
Corn, canned, cream style, white	1 cup	1	185	46	4	0	.2
Corn, canned, cream style, yellow	1 cup	1	185	46	4	0	.2
Corn, cooked from frozen, white	1 cup	0	135	34	5	0	0
Corn, cooked from frozen, white	1 ear	0	60	14	2	0	.1
Corn, cooked from frozen, yellow	1 cup	0	135	34	5	0	0
Corn, cooked from frozen, yellow	1 ear	0	60	14	2	0	.1
Corn, cooked from raw, white	1 ear	1	85	19	3	0	.2
Corn, cooked from raw, yellow	1 ear	1	85	19	3	0	.2
Corn, canned, whole kernel, white	1 cup	1	165	41	5	0	.2
Corn, canned, whole kernel, yellow	1 cup	1	165	41	5	0	.2
Cottage cheese, cr., large curd	1 cup	10	235	6	28	34	6.4
Cottage cheese, cr., w/fruit	1 cup	8	280	30	22	25	4.9
Cottage cheese, low-fat 2%	1 cup	4	205	8	31	19	2.8
Cottage cheese, uncreamed	1 cup	1	125	3	25	10	.4

Food Item	Amount	Fat Grams	Calories	Carbo Grams	Protein Grams	Chol. Mgs.	Saturated Fat
Cream of chicken soup w/water	1 cup	7	115	9	3	10	2.1
Cream of chicken soup w/milk	1 cup	11	190	15	7	27	4.6
Cream of mushroom soup w/water	1 cup	9	130	9	2	2	2.4
Cream of mushroom soup w/milk	1 cup	14	205	15	6	20	5.1
Crabmeat, canned	1 cup	3	135	1	23	135	.5
Cracked-wheat bread	1 slice	1	65	12	2	0	.2
Cranberry juice cocktail	1 cup	0	145	38	0	0	0
Cranberry sauce, canned, swtnd.	1 cup	0	420	108	1	0	0
Cream cheese	1 oz.	10	100	1	2	31	6.2
Cream of Wheat, cooked	1 pkt	0	100	21	3	0	0
Crème pie	1 piece	23	455	59	3	8	15
Creamed wheat, cooked	1 cup	0	140	29	4	0	.1
Croissants	1	12	235	27	5	13	3.5
Cucumber, w/peel	6 slices	0	5	1	0	0	0
Curry powder	1 tsp	0	5	1	0	0	0
Custard pie	1 piece	17	330	36	9	169	5.6
Custard, baked	1 cup	15	305	29	14	278	6.8
Dandelion, cooked, drained	1 cup	1	35	7	2	0	.1
Danish pastry, fruit	1	13	235	28	4	56	3.9
Danish pastry, plain, no nuts	1	12	220	26	4	49	3.6
Dates, chopped	1 cup	1	490	131	4	0	.3
Devil's Food Cake, frst., cupcake	1	4	120	20	2	19	1.8
Doughnuts, cake type, plain	1	12	210	24	3	20	2.8
Doughnuts, yeast-leavened, glazed	1	13	235	26	4	21	5.2
Duck, roasted, flesh only	1/2 duck	25	445	0	52	197	9.2
Eggnog	1 cup	19	340	34	10	149	11.3
Eggplant, cooked, steamed	1 cup	0	25	6	1	0	0
Eggs, cooked, fried	1	7	90	1	6	211	1.9
Eggs, cooked, hard-cooked	1	5	75	1	6	213	1.6
Eggs, cooked, poached	1	5	75	1	6	212	1.5
Eggs, cooked, scrambled/omelet	1	7	100	1	7	215	2.2
Eggs, raw, white	1	0	15	0	4	0	0
Eggs, raw, whole	1	5	75	1	6	213	1.6
Eggs, raw, yolk	1	5	60	0	3	213	1.6
Enchilada	1	6	235	24	20	19	7.7
Endive, curly, raw	1 cup	0	10	2	1	0	0
English muffin, egg, cheese, bacon	1	18	360	31	18	213	8
English muffins, plain	1	1	140	27	5	0	.3
Evaporated milk, skim, canned	1 cup	1	200	29	19	9	.3
Evaporated milk, whole, canned	1 cup	19	340	25	17	74	11.6
Fats, cooking/vegetable shortening	1 T	13	115	0	0	0	3.3
Feta cheese	1 oz.	6	75	1	4	25	4.2
Fig bars	4	4	210	42	2	27	1

Food Item	Amount	Fat Grams	Calories	Carbo Grams	Protein Grams	Chol. Mgs.	Saturated Fat
Figs, dried	10	2	475	122	6	0	.4
Filberts, (hazelnuts) chopped	1 cup	72	725	18	15	0	5.3
Fish sandwich, large, w/o cheese	1	27	470	41	18	91	6.3
Fish sandwich, regular, w/cheese	1	23	420	39	16	56	6.3
Fish sticks, frozen, reheated	1 stick	3	70	4	6	26	.8
Flounder or sole, baked, butter	3 oz.	6	120	0	16	68	3.2
Flounder or sole, baked, w/o fat	3 oz.	1	80	0	17	59	.3
Fondant, uncoated	1 oz.	0	105	27	0	0	0
Frankfurter, cooked	1	13	145	1	5	23	4.8
French bread	1 slice	1	100	18	3	0	.3
French salad dressing, low calorie	1 T	2	25	2	0	0	.2
French salad dressing, regular	1 T	9	85	1	0	0	1.4
French toast, home recipe	1 slice	7	155	17	6	112	1.6
Fried pie, apple	1 pie	14	255	31	2	14	5.8
Fried pie, cherry	1 pie	14	250	32	2	13	5.8
Froot Loops cereal	1 oz.	1	110	25	2	0	.2
Fruit cocktail, heavy syrup	1 cup	0	185	48	1	0	0
Fruit cocktail, juice packed	1 cup	0	115	29	1	0	0
Fruit punch drink, canned	6 F oz.	0	85	22	0	0	0
Fruitcake, dark, from home recipe	1 piece	7	165	25	2	20	1.5
Fudge, chocolate, plain	1 oz.	3	115	21	1	1	2.1
Garlic powder	1 tsp	0	10	2	0	0	0
Gelatin dessert, prepared	1/2 cup	0	70	17	2	0	0
Gelatin, dry	1 env.	0	25	0	6	0	0
Ginger ale	12 F oz.	0	125	32	0	0	0
Gingerbread cake, from mix	1 piece	4	175	32	2	1	1.1
Gin/rum/vodka/whiskey 80-proof	1.5 F oz.	0	95	0	0	0	0
Gin/rum/vodka/whiskey 90-proof	1.5 F oz.	0	110	0	0	0	0
Golden Grahams cereal	1 oz.	1	110	24	2	0	.7
Graham cracker, plain	2	1	60	11	1	0	.4
Grape-Nuts cereal	1 oz.	0	100	23	3	0	0
Grape drink, canned	6 F oz.	0	100	26	0	0	0
Grape juice, canned	1 cup	0	155	38	1	0	.1
Grape soda	12 F oz.	0	180	46	0	0	0
Grapefruit j., frzn., conc., unswten.	6 F oz.	1	300	72	4	0	.1
Grapefruit juice, canned, unswten.	1 cup	0	95	22	1	0	0
Grapefruit juice, raw	1 cup	0	95	23	1	0	0
Grapefruit, canned, syrup pack	1 cup	0	150	39	1	0	0
Grapefruit, raw, pink or white	1/2 fruit	0	40	10	1	0	0
Grape juice, frzn., conc., swten.	6 F oz.	1	385	96	1	0	.2
Grapes, European, raw, Thompson	10	0	35	9	0	0	.1
Gravy and turkey, frozen	5 oz.	4	95	7	8	26	1.2
Great northern beans, dry, cooked	1 cup	1	210	38	14	0	.1

Food Item	Amount	Fat Grams	Calories	Carbo Grams	Protein Grams	Chol. Mgs.	Saturated Fat
Ground beef, broiled, lean	3 oz.	16	230	0	21	74	6.2
Ground beef, broiled, regular	3 oz.	18	245	0	20	76	6.9
Gum drops	1 oz.	0	100	25	0	0	0
Haddock, breaded, fried	3 oz.	9	175	7	17	75	2.4
Half and half, cream	1 cup	28	315	10	7	89	17.3
Halibut, broiled, butter, lemon j.	3 oz.	6	140	0	20	62	3.3
Hamburger, 4 oz. patty	1	21	445	38	25	71	7.1
Hamburger, regular	1	11	245	28	12	32	4.4
Hard candy	1 oz.	0	110	28	0	0	0
Herring, pickled	3 oz.	13	190	0	17	85	4.3
Hollandaise sauce from mix	1 cup	20	240	14	5	52	11.6
Honey	1 T	0	65	17	0	0	0
Honey Nut Cheerios cereal	1 oz.	1	105	23	3	0	.1
Honeydew melon, raw	1/10	0	45	12	1	0	0
Ice cream, vanilla, regular 11% fat	1 cup	14	270	32	5	59	8.9
Ice cream, vanilla, rich 16% fat	1 cup	24	350	32	4	88	14.7
Ice cream, vanilla, soft serve	1 cup	23	375	38	7	153	13.5
Ice milk, vanilla, 4% fat	1 cup	6	185	29	5	18	3.5
Ice milk, vanilla, soft serve 3% fat	1 cup	5	225	38	8	13	2.9
Imitation creamers, liquid frozen	1 T	1	20	2	0	0	1.4
Imitation creamers, powdered	1 tsp	1	10	1	0	0	.7
Imitation whipped topping, frz.	1 T	1	15	1	0	0	.9
Imitation sour dressing	1 T	2	20	1	0	1	1.6
Imitation whipped topping	1 T	1	10	1	0	0	.8
Italian bread	1 slice	0	85	17	3	0	0
Italian salad dressing, low calorie	1 T	0	5	2	0	0	0
Italian salad dressing, regular	1 T	9	80	1	0	0	1.3
Jams and preserves	1 T	0	55	14	0	0	0
Jellies	1 T	0	50	13	0	0	0
Jelly beans	1 oz.	0	105	26	0	0	0
Jerusalem-artichoke, raw	1 cup	0	115	26	3	0	0
Kale, cooked from frozen	1 cup	1	40	7	4	0	.1
Kale, cooked from raw	1 cup	1	40	7	2	0	.1
Kiwifruit, raw	1	0	45	11	1	0	0
Kohlrabi, cooked, drained	1 cup	0	50	11	3	0	0
Lamb, rib, roasted, lean only	2 oz.	7	130	0	15	50	3.2
Lamb, chops, arm, braised, lean	1.7 oz.	7	135	0	17	59	2.9
Lamb, chops, loin, broil, lean	2.3 oz.	6	140	0	19	60	2.6
Lamb, leg, roasted, lean only	2.6 oz.	6	140	0	20	65	2.4
Lard	1 T	13	115	0	0	12	5.1
Lemon-lime soda	12 F oz.	0	155	39	0	0	0
Lemon juice, canned	1 T	0	5	1	0	0	0
Lemon juice, raw	1 cup	0	60	21	1	0	0

Food Item	Amount	Fat Grams	Calories	Carbo Grams	Protein Grams	Chol. Mgs.	Saturated Fat
Lemon juice, frzn., single-strength	6 F oz.	1	55	16	1	0	.1
Lemon meringue pie	1 piece	14	355	53	5	143	4.3
Lemonade, concentrate, fzn., undil.	6 F oz.	0	425	112	0	0	0
Lemons, raw	1 lemon	0	15	5	1	0	0
Lentils, dry, cooked	1 cup	1	215	38	16	0	.1
Lettuce, butterhead, raw, head	1 head	0	20	4	2	0	0
Lettuce, crisphead, raw, head	1 head	1	70	11	5	0	.1
Lettuce, crisphead, raw, pieces	1 cup	0	5	1	1	0	0
Lettuce, looseleaf	1 cup	0	10	2	1	0	0
Light, coffee or table cream	1 T	3	30	1	0	10	1.8
Lima beans, dry, cooked	1 cup	1	260	49	16	0	.2
Lima beans, baby, frzn., ckd.	1 cup	1	190	35	12	0	.1
Lima beans, thick seed, frzn., ckd.	1 cup	1	170	32	10	0	.1
Lime juice, raw	1 cup	0	65	22	1	0	0
Lime juice, canned	1 cup	1	50	16	1	0	.1
Limeade, concentrate, frzn., undil.	6 F oz.	0	410	108	0	0	0
Lucky Charms cereal	1 oz.	1	110	23	3	0	.2
Macadamia nuts, oil roasted	1 oz.	22	205	4	2	0	3.2
Macaroni and cheese, canned	1 cup	10	230	26	9	24	4.7
Macaroni and cheese, home recipe	1 cup	22	430	40	17	44	9.8
Macaroni, cooked, firm	1 cup	1	190	39	7	0	.1
Malt-O-Meal	1 cup	0	120	26	4	0	0
Malted milk, chocolate, powder	3/4 oz.	1	85	18	1	1	.5
Malted milk, natural, powder	3/4 oz.	2	85	15	3	4	.9
Mangos, raw	1	1	135	35	1	0	.1
Margarine, imitation 40% fat	1 T	5	50	0	0	0	1.1
Margarine, regular, hard, 80% fat	1 T	11	100	0	0	0	2.2
Margarine, regular, soft, 80% fat	1 T	11	100	0	0	0	1.9
Margarine, spread, hard, 60% fat	1 T	9	75	0	0	0	2
Margarine, spread, soft, 60% fat	1 T	9	75	0	0	0	1.8
Marshmallows	1 oz.	0	90	23	1	0	0
Mayonnaise type salad dressing	1 T	5	60	4	0	4	.7
Mayonnaise, regular	1 T	11	100	0	0	8	1.7
Melba toast, plain	1 piece	0	20	4	1	0	.1
Milk chocolate candy, plain	1 oz.	9	145	16	2	6	5.4
Milk chocolate candy, w/almond	1 oz.	10	150	15	3	5	4.8
Milk chocolate candy, w/peanuts	1 oz.	11	155	13	4	5	4.2
Milk chocolate candy, w/rice crpy.	1 oz.	7	140	18	2	6	4.4
Milk, low-fat, 1%, no added solid	1 cup	3	100	12	8	10	1.6
Milk, low-fat, 2%, no added solid	1 cup	5	120	12	8	18	2.9
Milk, skim, no added milk solid	1 cup	0	85	12	8	4	.3
Milk, whole, 3.3% fat	1 cup	8	150	11	8	33	5.1
Minestrone soup, canned	1 cup	3	80	11	4	2	.6

Food Item	Amount	Fat Grams	Calories	Carbo Grams	Protein Grams	Chol. Mgs.	Saturated Fat
Miso soup	1 cup	13	470	65	29	0	1.8
Mixed grain bread	1 slice	1	65	12	2	0	.2
Mixed nuts w/peanuts, dry	1 oz.	15	170	7	5	0	2
Mixed nuts w/peanuts, oil	1 oz.	16	175	6	5	0	2.5
Molasses, cane, blackstrap	2 T	0	85	22	0	0	0
Mozzarella cheese, whole milk	1 oz.	6	80	1	6	22	3.7
Mozzarella cheese, skim, lo-moist.	1 oz.	5	80	1	8	15	3.1
Muenster cheese	1 oz.	9	105	0	7	27	5.4
Mushroom gravy, canned	1 cup	6	120	13	3	0	1
Mushrooms, canned	1 cup	0	35	8	3	0	.1
Mushrooms, cooked	1 cup	1	40	8	3	0	.1
Mushrooms, raw	1 cup	0	20	3	1	0	0
Mustard greens, cooked	1 cup	0	20	3	3	0	0
Mustard, prepared, yellow	1 tsp	0	5	0	0	0	0
Nature Valley Granola cereal	1 oz.	5	125	19	3	0	3.3
Nectarines, raw	1	1	65	16	1	0	.1
Nonfat dry milk, instantized	1 cup	0	245	35	24	12	.3
Nonfat dry milk, instantized	1 env.	1	325	47	32	17	.4
Noodles, chow mein, canned	1 cup	11	220	26	6	5	2.1
Noodles, egg, cooked	1 cup	2	200	37	7	50	.5
Oatmeal bread	1 slice	1	65	12	2	0	.2
Oatmeal w/raisins cookies	4	10	245	36	3	2	2.5
Oatmeal, cooked, flavored, instant	1 pkt	2	160	31	5	0	.3
Oatmeal, cooked, plain, instant	1 pkt	2	105	18	4	0	.3
Oatmeal, cooked, rg., qck., instant	1 cup	2	145	25	6	0	.4
Ocean perch, breaded, fried	1 fillet	11	185	7	16	66	2.6
Okra pods, cooked	8 pods	0	25	6	2	0	0
Olive oil	1 cup	216	1910	0	0	0	29.2
Olive oil	1 T	14	125	0	0	0	1.9
Olives, canned, green	4 med.	2	15	0	0	0	.2
Olives, canned, ripe, mission	3 small	2	15	0	0	0	.3
Onion powder	1 tsp	0	5	2	0	0	0
Onion rings, breaded, frozen	2 rings	5	80	8	1	0	1.7
Onion soup, dehydrated	1 pkt	0	20	4	1	0	.1
Onions, raw, chopped	1 cup	0	55	12	2	0	.1
Onions, raw, cooked, drained	1 cup	0	60	13	2	0	.1
Onions, raw, sliced	1 cup	0	40	8	1	0	.1
Onions, spring, raw	6	0	10	2	1	0	0
Orange juice, canned	1 cup	0	105	25	1	0	0
Orange juice, raw	1 cup	0	110	26	2	0	.1
Orange juice, frozen, concentrate	6 F oz.	0	340	81	5	0	.1
Orange juice, frozen, concentrate	1 cup	0	110	27	2	0	0
Orange soda	12 F oz.	0	180	46	0	0	0

Food Item	Amount	Fat Grams	Calories	Carbo Grams	Protein Grams	Chol. Mgs.	Saturated Fat
Orange + grapefruit juice, canned	1 cup	0	105	25	1	0	0
Oranges, raw	1	0	60	15	1	0	0
Oranges, raw, sections	1 cup	0	85	21	2	0	0
Oregano	1 tsp	0	5	1	0	0	0
Oysters, breaded, fried	1 oyster	5	90	5	5	35	1.4
Oysters, raw	1 cup	4	160	8	20	120	1.4
Pancakes, buckwheat	1	2	55	6	2	20	.9
Pancakes, plain	1	2	60	9	2	16	.5
Papayas, raw	1 cup	0	65	17	1	0	.1
Paprika	1 tsp	0	5	1	0	0	0
Parmesan cheese, grated	1 cup	30	455	4	42	79	19.1
Parmesan cheese, grated	1 oz.	9	130	1	12	22	5.4
Parmesan cheese, grated	1 T	2	25	0	2	4	1
Parsley, freeze-dried	1 T	0	0	0	0	0	0
Parsley, raw	10 sprig	0	5	1	0	0	0
Parsnips, cooked, drained	1 cup	0	125	30	2	0	.1
Pasteurized process cheese, Swiss	1 oz.	7	95	1	7	24	4.5
Pasteurized proc. cheese, American	1 oz.	9	105	0	6	27	5.6
Pasteurized proc. ch. spread, Am.	1 oz.	6	80	2	5	16	3.8
Pea beans, dry, cooked	1 cup	1	225	40	15	0	.1
Peach pie	1 piece	17	405	60	4	0	4.1
Peaches, canned, heavy syrup	1 cup	0	190	51	1	0	0
Peaches, canned, heavy syrup	1 half	0	60	16	0	0	0
Peaches, canned, juice pack	1 cup	0	110	29	2	0	0
Peaches, canned, juice pack	1 half	0	35	9	0	0	0
Peaches, dried	1 cup	1	380	98	6	0	.1
Peaches, dried, cooked, unsweet.	1 cup	1	200	51	3	0	.1
Peaches, frozen, sweetened	1 cup	0	235	60	2	0	0
Peaches, frozen, sweetened	10 oz.	0	265	68	2	0	0
Peaches, raw	1	0	35	10	1	0	0
Peaches, raw, sliced	1 cup	0	75	19	1	0	0
Peanut butter	1 T	8	95	3	5	0	1.4
Peanut butter cookie	4	14	245	28	4	22	4
Peanut oil	1 cup	216	1910	0	0	0	36.5
Peanut oil	1 T	14	125	0	0	0	2.4
Peanuts, oil roasted	1 cup	71	840	27	39	0	9.9
Peanuts, oil roasted	1 oz.	14	165	5	8	0	1.9
Pears, canned, heavy syrup	1 cup	0	190	49	1	0	0
Pears, canned, heavy syrup	1 half	0	60	15	0	0	0
Pears, canned, juice pack	1 cup	0	125	32	1	0	0
Pears, canned, juice pack	1 half	0	40	10	0	0	0
Pears, raw, bartlett	1	1	100	25	1	0	0
Pears, raw, bosc	1	1	85	21	1	0	0

Food Item	Amount	Fat Grams	Calories	Carbo Grams	Protein Grams	Chol. Mgs.	Saturated Fat
Pears, raw, d'anjou	1	1	120	30	1	0	0
Peas, edible pod, cooked	1 cup	0	65	11	5	0	.1
Peas, green, canned	1 cup	1	115	21	8	0	.1
Peas, split, dry, cooked	1 cup	1	230	42	16	0	.1
Peas, green, frozen, cooked	1 cup	0	125	23	8	0	.1
Pea, green, soup, canned	1 cup	3	165	27	9	0	1.4
Pecan pie	1 piece	32	575	71	7	95	4.7
Pecans, halves	1 cup	73	720	20	8	0	5.9
Pecans, halves	1 oz.	19	190	5	2	0	1.5
Peppers, hot chili, raw, red or gr.	1	0	20	4	1	0	0
Peppers, sweet, cooked, red or gr.	1	0	15	3	0	0	0
Peppers, sweet, raw, red or green	1	0	20	4	1	0	0
Pepper, black	1 tsp	0	5	1	0	0	0
Pickles, cucumber, dill	1	0	5	1	0	0	0
Pickles, cucumber, fresh pack	2 slices	0	10	3	0	0	0
Pickles, cucumber, swt. Gherkin	1 pickle	0	20	5	0	0	0
Pie crust from mix	2 crust	93	1485	141	20	0	22.7
Pie crust from home recipe	1 shell	60	900	79	11	0	14.8
Pine nuts	1 oz.	17	160	5	3	0	2.7
Pineapple-grapefruit juice drink	6 F oz.	0	90	23	0	0	0
Pineapple, canned, unsweetened	1 cup	0	140	34	1	0	0
Pineapple, canned, heavy syrup	1 cup	0	200	52	1	0	0
Pineapple, canned, heavy syrup	1 slice	0	45	12	0	0	0
Pineapple, canned, juice pack	1 cup	0	150	39	1	0	0
Pineapple, canned, juice pack	1 slice	0	35	9	0	0	0
Pineapple, raw, diced	1 cup	1	75	19	1	0	0
Pinto beans, dry, cooked, drained	1 cup	1	265	49	15	0	.1
Pistachio nuts	1 oz.	14	165	7	6	0	1.7
Pita bread	1 pita	1	165	33	6	0	.1
Pizza, cheese	1 slice	9	290	39	15	56	4.1
Plantains, cooked	1 cup	0	180	48	1	0	.1
Plantains, raw	1	1	220	57	2	0	.3
Plums, canned, heavy syrup	1 cup	0	230	60	1	0	0
Plums, canned, juice pack	1 cup	0	145	38	1	0	0
Plums, raw, 1-1/2" diameter	1	0	15	4	0	0	0
Plums, raw, 2-1/8" diameter	1	0	35	9	1	0	0
Popcorn, air-popped, unsalted	1 cup	0	30	6	1	0	0
Popcorn, popped, veg., oil, salted	1 cup	3	55	6	1	0	.5
Popcorn, sugar syrup coated	1 cup	1	135	30	2	0	.1
Popsicle	1	0	70	18	0	0	0
Pork chop, loin, broil, lean	2.5 oz.	8	165	0	23	71	2.6
Pork chop, loin, broil, lean + fat	3.1 oz.	19	275	0	24	84	7
Pork chop, loin, panfry, lean	2.4 oz.	11	180	0	19	72	3.7

Food Item	Amount	Fat Grams	Calories	Carbo Grams	Protein Grams	Chol. Mgs.	Saturated Fat
Pork chop, loin, panfry, lean + fat	3.1 oz.	27	335	0	21	92	9.8
Pork fresh ham, roasted, lean	2.5 oz.	8	160	0	20	68	2.7
Pork fresh ham, roasted, lean + fat	3 oz.	18	250	0	21	79	6.4
Pork fresh rib, roasted, lean	2.5 oz.	10	175	0	20	56	3.4
Pork fresh rib, roasted, lean + fat	3 oz.	20	270	0	21	69	7.2
Pork shoulder, braised, lean	2.4 oz.	8	165	0	22	76	2.8
Pork shoulder, braised, lean + fat	3 oz.	22	295	0	23	93	7.9
Pork, cured, bacon, reg., cooked	3 slice	9	110	0	6	16	3.3
Pork, cured, can. bacon, cooked	2 slice	4	85	1	11	27	1.3
Pork, cured, ham, canned, roast	3 oz.	7	140	0	18	35	2.4
Pork, cured, ham, roasted, lean	2.4 oz.	4	105	0	17	37	1.3
Pork, link, cooked	1 link	4	50	0	3	11	1.4
Pork, luncheon meat, canned	2 slices	13	140	1	5	26	4.5
Pork, luncheon meat, chopped ham	2 slices	7	95	0	7	21	2.4
Pork, luncheon meat, ckd. ham	2 slices	6	105	2	10	32	1.9
Potato chips	10 chips	7	105	10	1	0	1.8
Potato salad with mayonnaise	1 cup	21	360	28	7	170	3.6
Potatoes, au gratin, from mix	1 cup	10	230	31	6	12	6.3
Potatoes, baked w/o skin	1 potato	0	145	34	3	0	0
Potatoes, baked with skin	1 potato	0	220	51	5	0	.1
Potatoes, boiled	1 potato	0	115	27	2	0	0
Potatoes, hashed brown	1 cup	18	340	44	5	0	7
Potatoes, mashed, from dehydrated	1 cup	12	235	32	4	29	7.2
Potatoes, mash., rec., w/milk/mar.	1 cup	9	225	35	4	4	2.2
Potatoes, mashed, recipe, w/milk	1 cup	1	160	37	4	4	.7
Potatoes, scalloped, from mix	1 cup	11	230	31	5	27	6.5
Potatoes, French fried, frozen, fried	10	8	160	20	2	0	2.5
Potatoes, French fried, frozen, oven	10	4	110	17	2	0	2.1
Pound cake	1 slice	5	110	15	2	64	3
Pretzels, stick	10	0	10	2	0	0	0
Pretzels, twisted, Dutch	1	1	65	13	2	0	.1
Pretzels, twisted, thin	10	2	240	48	6	0	.4
Product 19 cereal	1 oz.	0	110	24	3	0	0
Provolene cheese	1 oz.	8	100	1	7	20	4.8
Prune juice, canned	1 cup	0	180	45	2	0	0
Prunes, dried	5	0	115	31	1	0	0
Prunes, dried, cooked, unsweetened	1 cup	0	225	60	2	0	0
Pudding, chocolate, canned	5 oz.	11	205	30	3	1	9.5
Pudding, choc., cooked from mix	1/2 cup	4	150	25	4	15	2.4
Pudding, choc., instant from mix	1/2 cup	4	155	27	4	14	2.3
Pudding, rice, from mix	1/2 cup	4	155	27	4	15	2.3
Pudding, tapioca, canned	5 oz.	5	160	28	3	0	4.8
Pudding, tapioca, from mix	1/2 cup	4	145	25	4	15	2.3

Food Item	Amount	Fat Grams	Calories	Carbo Grams	Protein Grams	Chol. Mgs.	Saturated Fat
Pudding, vanilla, canned	5 oz.	10	220	33	2	1	9.5
Pudding, vanilla, cooked from mix	1/2 cup	4	145	25	4	15	2.3
Pudding, vanilla, instant	1/2 cup	4	150	27	4	15	2.2
Pumpernickel bread	1 slice	1	80	16	3	0	.2
Pumpkin and squash kernels	1 oz.	13	155	5	7	0	2.5
Pumpkin pie	1 slice	17	320	37	6	109	6.4
Pumpkin, canned	1 cup	1	85	20	3	0	.4
Pumpkin, cooked	1 cup	0	50	12	2	0	.1
Quiche Lorraine	1 slice	48	600	29	13	285	23.2
Radishes, raw	4	0	5	1	0	0	0
Raisin Bran, Kellogg's	1 oz	1	90	21	3	0	.1
Raisin Bran, Post	1 oz.	1	85	21	3	0	.1
Raisin bread	1 slice	1	65	13	2	0	.2
Raisins	1 cup	1	435	115	5	0	.2
Raspberries, frozen, sweetened	1 cup	0	255	65	2	0	0
Raspberries, frozen, sweetened	10 oz.	0	295	74	2	0	0
Raspberries, raw	1 cup	1	60	14	1	0	0
Red kidney beans, dry, canned	1 cup	1	230	42	15	0	.1
Refried, beans, canned	1 cup	3	295	51	18	0	.4
Relish, sweet	1 T	0	20	5	0	0	0
Rhubarb, cooked, added sugar	1 cup	0	280	75	1	0	0
Rice Krispies cereal	1 oz.	0	110	25	2	0	0
Rice, brown, cooked	1 cup	1	230	50	5	0	.3
Rice, white, cooked	1 cup	0	225	50	4	0	.1
Rice, white, instant, cooked	1 cup	0	180	40	4	0	.1
Rice, white, parboiled, cooked	1 cup	0	185	41	4	0	0
Rice, white, parboiled, raw	1 cup	1	685	150	14	0	.1
Rice, white, raw	1 cup	1	670	149	12	0	.2
Ricotta cheese, skim milk	1 cup	19	340	13	28	76	12.1
Ricotta cheese, whole milk	1 cup	32	430	7	28	124	20.4
Roast beef sandwich	1	13	345	34	22	55	3.5
Rolls, dinner	1	2	85	14	2	0	.5
Rolls, frankfurter or hamburger	1	2	115	20	3	0	.5
Rolls, hard	1	2	155	30	5	0	.4
Rolls, hoagie or submarine	1	8	400	72	11	0	1.8
Root beer	12 F oz.	0	165	42	0	0	0
Rye bread, light	1 slice	1	65	12	2	0	.2
Rye wafers, whole-grain	2	1	55	10	1	0	.3
Safflower oil	1 cup	218	1925	0	0	0	19.8
Safflower oil	1 T	14	125	0	0	0	1.3
Salami, cooked type	2 slices	11	145	1	8	37	4.6
Salami, dry type	2 slices	7	85	1	5	16	2.4
Salmon, baked, red	3 oz.	5	140	0	21	60	1.2

Food Item	Amount	Fat Grams	Calories	Carbo Grams	Protein Grams	Chol. Mgs.	Saturated Fat
Salmon, canned, pink, w/bones	3 oz.	5	120	0	17	34	.9
Salmon, smoked	3 oz.	8	150	0	18	51	2.6
Saltines	4	1	50	9	1	4	.5
Sandwich spread, pork, beef	1 T	3	35	2	1	6	.9
Sandwich type cookie	4	8	195	29	2	0	2
Sardines, Atlantic, canned, oil, dr.	3 oz.	9	175	0	20	85	2.1
Sauerkraut, canned	1 cup	0	45	10	2	0	.1
Scallops, breaded, frozen, reheat	6	10	195	10	15	70	2.5
Seaweed, kelp, raw	1 oz.	0	10	3	0	0	.1
Seaweed, spirulina, dried	1 oz.	2	80	7	16	0	.8
Self-rising flour	1 cup	1	440	93	12	0	.2
Semisweet chocolate	1 cup	61	860	97	7	0	36.2
Sesame seeds	1 T	4	45	1	2	0	.6
Shakes, chocolate, thick	10 oz.	8	335	60	9	30	4.8
Shakes, vanilla, thick	10 oz.	9	315	50	11	33	5.3
Sheetcake, with frosting home rec.	1 piece	14	445	77	4	70	4.6
Sheetcake, w/o frosting home rec.	1 piece	12	315	48	4	61	3.3
Sherbet, 2% fat	1 cup	4	270	59	2	14	2.4
Shortbread cookie	4	8	155	20	2	27	2.9
Shredded Wheat cereal	1 oz.	1	100	23	3	0	.1
Shrimp, canned, drained	3 oz.	1	100	1	21	128	.2
Shrimp, French fried	3 oz.	10	200	11	16	168	2.5
Snack type crackers	1	1	15	2	0	0	.2
Snap bean, canned or frozen, dr.	1 cup	0	25	6	2	0	0
Snap bean, raw, cooked, drained	1 cup	0	45	10	2	0	.1
Sour cream	1 cup	48	495	10	7	102	30
Sour cream	1 T	3	25	1	0	5	1.6
Soy sauce	1 T	0	10	2	2	0	0
Soybean-cottonseed oil, hydr.	1 cup	218	1925	0	0	0	39.2
Soybean-cottonseed oil, hydr.	1 T	14	125	0	0	0	2.5
Soybean oil, hydrogenated	1 cup	218	1925	0	0	0	32.5
Soybean oil, hydrogenated	1 T	14	125	0	0	0	2.1
Soybeans, dry, cooked, drained	1 cup	10	235	19	20	0	1.3
Spaghetti, cooked, firm	1 cup	1	190	39	7	0	.1
Spaghetti, cooked, tender	1 cup	1	155	32	5	0	.1
Spaghetti, tom. sauce & cheese	1 cup	2	190	39	6	3	.4
Spaghetti and meatballs	1 cup	12	330	39	19	89	3.9
Special K Cereal	1 oz.	0	110	21	6	0	0
Spinach soufflé	1 cup	18	220	3	11	184	7.1
Spinach, canned, drained	1 cup	1	50	7	6	0	.2
Spinach, cooked	1 cup	0	40	7	5	0	.1
Spinach, raw	1 cup	0	10	2	2	0	0
Squash, summer, cooked	1 cup	1	35	8	2	0	.1

Food Item	Amount	Fat Grams	Calories	Carbo Grams	Protein Grams	Chol. Mgs.	Saturated Fat
Squash, winter, baked	1 cup	1	80	18	2	0	.3
Strawberries, frozen, sweetened	1 cup	0	245	66	1	0	0
Strawberries, frozen, sweetened	10 oz.	0	275	74	2	0	0
Strawberries, raw	1 cup	1	45	10	1	0	0
Sugar cookie, from ref. dough	4	12	235	31	2	29	2.3
Sugar Frosted Flakes, Kellogg's	1 oz.	0	110	26	1	0	0
Sugar Smacks cereal	1 oz.	1	105	25	2	0	.1
Sugar, brown	1 cup	0	820	212	0	0	0
Sugar, powdered	1	0	385	100	0	0	0
Sugar, white, granulated	1 cup	0	770	199	0	0	0
Sugar, white, granulated	1 pkt	0	25	6	0	0	0
Sugar, white, granulated	1 T	0	45	12	0	0	0
Sunflower oil	1 cup	218	1925	0	0	0	22.5
Sunflower oil	1 T	14	125	0	0	0	1.4
Sunflower seeds	1 oz.	14	160	5	6	0	1.5
Sweet (dark) chocolate	1 oz.	10	150	16	1	0	5.9
Sweetened condensed milk	1 cup	27	980	166	24	104	16.8
Sweet potatoes, baked, peeled	1	0	115	28	2	0	0
Sweet potatoes, candied	1 piece	3	145	29	1	8	1.4
Sweet potatoes, canned, mashed	1 cup	1	260	59	5	0	.1
Swiss cheese	1 oz.	8	105	1	8	26	5
Syrup, chocolate flavor, fudge	2 T	5	125	21	2	0	3.1
Table syrup (corn and maple)	2 T	0	122	32	0	0	0
Taco	1	11	195	15	9	21	4.1
Tahini	1 T	8	90	3	3	0	1.1
Tangerine juice, canned, sweet.	1 cup	0	125	30	1	0	0
Tangerines, canned, light syrup	1 cup	0	155	41	1	0	0
Tangerines, raw	1	0	35	9	1	0	0
Tartar sauce	1 T	8	75	1	0	4	1.2
Tea, brewed	8 F oz.	0	0	0	0	0	0
Tea, instant, unsweetened	8 F oz.	0	0	1	0	0	0
Tea, instant, sweetened	8 F oz.	0	85	22	0	0	0
Tofu	1 piece	5	85	3	9	0	.7
Tomato juice	1 cup	0	40	10	2	0	0
Tomato paste, canned	1 cup	2	220	49	10	0	.3
Tomato puree, canned	1 cup	0	105	25	4	0	0
Tomato sauce, canned	1 cup	0	75	18	3	0	.1
Tomato soup, w/milk, canned	1 cup	6	160	22	6	17	2.9
Tomato soup, w/water, canned	1 cup	2	85	17	2	0	.4
Tomato veg. soup, dehydrated	1 pkt.	1	40	8	1	0	.3
Tomatoes, canned	1 cup	1	50	10	2	0	.1
Tomatoes, raw	1	0	25	5	1	0	0
Tortillas, corn	1	1	65	13	2	0	.1

Food Item	Amount	Fat Grams	Calories	Carbo Grams	Protein Grams	Chol. Mgs.	Saturated Fat
Total cereal	1 oz.	1	100	22	3	0	.1
Trix cereal	1 oz.	0	110	25	2	0	.2
Trout, broiled w/butter/lemon	3 oz.	9	175	0	21	71	4.1
Tuna salad	1 cup	19	375	19	33	80	3.3
Tuna, light, can., drained, water	3 oz.	7	165	0	24	55	1.4
Tuna, white, can., drained, water	3 oz.	1	135	0	30	48	.3
Turkey, dark w/o skin	4 oz.	8.2	212	0	32.4	96	-
Turkey, light w/o skin	4 oz.	3.7	178	0	33.9	78	-
Turnip greens, cooked	1 cup	0	30	6	2	0	.1
Turnips, cooked, diced	1 cup	0	30	8	1	0	0
Vanilla wafers	10	7	185	29	2	25	1.8
Veal cutlet, medium fat	3 oz.	9	185	0	23	86	4.1
Veal rib, medium fat, roasted	3 oz.	14	230	0	23	109	6
Vegetable beef soup, canned	1 cup	2	80	10	6	5	.9
Vegetable juice cocktail, canned	1 cup	0	45	11	2	0	0
Vegetables, mixed, canned	1 cup	0	75	15	4	0	.1
Vegetables, mixed, frozen	1 cup	0	105	24	5	0	.1
Vegetarian soup	1 cup	2	70	12	2	0	.3
Vienna bread	1 slice	1	70	13	2	0	.2
Vienna sausage	1	4	45	0	2	8	1.5
Vinegar and oil salad dressing	1 T	8	70	0	0	0	1.5
Vinegar, cider	1 T	0	0	1	0	0	0
Waffles, from mix	1	8	205	27	7	59	2.7
Walnuts, black, chopped	1 cup	71	760	15	30	0	4.5
Walnuts, black, chopped	1 oz.	16	170	3	7	0	1
Water chestnuts, canned	1 cup	0	70	17	1	0	0
Watermelon, raw	1 piece	2	155	35	3	0	.3
Watermelon, raw, diced	1 cup	1	50	11	1	0	.1
Wheat bread	1 slice	1	65	12	2	0	.2
Wheat flour, all-purpose	1 cup	1	420	88	12	0	.2
Wheaties cereal	1 oz.	0	100	23	3	0	.1
Wheat, thin crackers	4	1	35	5	1	0	.5
Whipped cream, unwhipped heavy	1 cup	88	820	7	5	326	54.8
Whipped cream, unwhipped light	1 cup	74	700	7	5	265	46.2
White bread	1 slice	1	65	12	2	0	.3
White bread crumbs	1 cup	2	120	22	4	0	.6
White cake, w/frosting	1 piece	9	260	42	3	3	2.1
White sauce, w/milk from mix	1 cup	13	240	21	10	34	6.4
Whole-wheat bread	1 slice	1	70	13	3	0	.4
Whole-wheat flour	1 cup	2	400	85	16	0	.3
Whole-wheat wafer/crackers	2	2	35	5	1	0	.5
Wine cooler	12 F oz.	0	190	29	0	0	0
Wine, dessert	3.5 F oz.	0	140	8	0	0	0

Food Item	Amount	Fat Grams	Calories	Carbo Grams	Protein Grams	Chol. Mgs.	Saturated Fat
Wine, table, red	3.5 F oz.	0	75	3	0	0	0
Wine, table, white	3.5 F oz.	0	80	3	0	0	0
Yeast, baker's, dry active	1 pkg.	0	20	3	3	0	0
Yellow cake w/choc. frosting	1 piece	8	235	40	3	36	3
Yogurt, w/low-fat milk	8 oz.	4	145	16	12	14	2.3
Yogurt, w/nonfat milk	8 oz.	0	125	17	13	4	.3
Yogurt, w/whole milk	8 oz.	7	140	11	8	29	4.8

Food Item	Amount	Total Calories	Fat Calories	Total Fat (g)	Sat. Fat (g)	Chol. (mg)	Sodium (mg)	Carbo (g)	Protein (g)
Arby's®									
Roast Beef Sandwiches									
Melt w/Cheddar	1	340	139	15	5	70	890	36	16
Arby-Q	1	360	130	14	4	70	1530	40	16
Beef 'N Cheddar	1	480	221	24	8	90	1240	43	23
Big Montana	1	630	290	32	15	155	2080	41	47
Giant Roast Beef	1	480	206	23	10	110	1440	41	32
Junior Roast Beef	1	310	121	13	4.5	70	740	34	16
Regular Roast Beef	1	350	151	16	6	85	950	34	21
Super Roast Beef	1	470	207	23	7	85	1130	47	22
Other Sandwiches									
Chicken Bacon 'N Swiss	1	610	293	33	8	110	1550	49	31
Chicken Breast Fillet	1	540	265	30	5	90	1160	47	24
Chicken Cordon Bleu	1	630	309	35	8	120	1820	47	34
Grilled Chicken Deluxe	1	450	198	22	4	110	1050	37	29
Roast Chicken Club	1	520	260	28	7	115	1440	38	29
Hot Ham 'N Swiss	1	340	119	13	4.5	90	1450	35	23
Sub Sandwiches									
French Dip	1	440	158	18	8	100	1680	42	28
Hot Ham 'N Swiss	1	530	239	27	8	110	1860	45	29
Italian	1	780	468	53	15	120	2440	49	29
Philly Beef 'N Swiss	1	700	378	42	15	130	1940	46	36
Roast Beef	1	760	426	48	16	130	2230	47	35
Turkey	1	630	328	37	9	100	2170	51	26
Market Fresh Sandwiches									
Roast Beef & Swiss	1	810	381	42	13	130	1780	73	37
Roast Ham & Swiss	1	730	307	34	8	125	2180	74	36
Roast Chicken Caesar	1	820	336	38	9	140	2160	75	43
Roast Turkey & Swiss	1	760	296	33	6	130	1920	75	43
Market Fresh Salads (dressing not included)									
Turkey Club Salad	1	350	189	21	10	90	920	9	33
Caesar Salad	1	90	34	4	2.5	10	170	8	7
Grilled Chicken Caesar	1	230	69	8	3.5	80	920	8	33
Chicken Finger Salad	1	570	308	34	9	65	1300	39	30
Caesar Side Salad	1	45	20	2	1	5	95	4	4

Food Item	Amount	Total Calories	Fat Calories	Total Fat (g)	Sat. Fat (g)	Chol. (mg)	Sodium (mg)	Carbo (g)	Protein (g)
Light Menu									
Light Grilled Chicken	1	280	48	5	1.5	55	1170	30	29
Lt Roast Chicken Deluxe	1	260	44	5	1	40	1010	33	23
Lt Roast Turkey Deluxe	1	260	44	5	0.5	40	980	33	23
Roast Chicken Salad	1	160	21	2.5	0	40	700	15	20
Grilled Chicken Salad	1	210	40	4.5	1.5	65	800	14	30
Garden Salad	1	70	5	1	0	0	45	14	4
Side Salad	1	25	0	0	0	0	20	5	2
Side Items									
Cheddar Curly Fries	1	460	221	24	6	5	1290	54	6
Curly Fries (small)	1	310	140	15	3.5	0	770	39	4
Curly Fries (medium)	1	400	180	20	5	0	990	50	5
Curly Fries (large)	1	620	273	30	7	0	1540	78	8
Homestyle Fries (child)	1	220	86	10	2.5	0	430	32	3
Homestyle Fries (small)	1	300	120	13	3.5	0	570	42	3
Homestyle Fries (med.)	1	370	141	16	4	0	710	53	4
Homestyle Fries (large)	1	560	218	24	6	0	1070	79	6
Potato Cakes	2	250	140	16	4	0	490	26	2
Jalapeno Bites	1	330	188	21	9	40	670	30	7
Mozzarella Sticks	4	470	259	29	14	60	1330	34	18
Onion Petals	1	410	221	24	3.5	0	300	43	4
Chicken Finger Snack	1	580	290	32	7	35	1450	55	19
Chicken Finger 4-Pack	1	640	352	38	8	70	1590	42	31
Baked Pot. w/Btr/Sr Crm	1	500	210	24	15	55	170	65	8
Broccoli 'N Cheddar BP	1	540	211	24	12	50	680	71	12
Deluxe Baked Potato	1	650	312	34	20	90	750	67	20
Desserts									
Iced Apple Turnover	1	420	139	16	4.5	0	230	65	4
Cherry Turnover	1	410	139	16	4.5	0	250	63	4
Breakfast Items									
Biscuit w/Butter	1	280	151	17	4	0	780	27	5
Biscuit w/Ham	1	330	182	20	5	30	830	28	12
Biscuit w/Sausage	1	460	299	33	9	25	300	28	12
Biscuit w/Bacon	1	360	220	24	7	10	220	27	9
Croissant w/Ham	1	310	171	19	11	50	1130	29	13
Croissant w/Sausage	1	440	290	32	15	45	600	29	13
Croissant w/Bacon	1	340	211	23	13	30	520	28	10
Sourdough w/Ham	1	390	47	6	1	30	1570	67	19
Sourdough w/Sausage	1	520	172	19	5	25	1040	67	19
Sourdough w/Bacon	1	420	88	10	2.5	10	960	66	16
French Toastix (no syrup)	1	370	152	17	4	0	440	48	7

Food Item	Amount	Total Calories	Fat Calories	Total Fat (g)	Sat. Fat (g)	Chol. (mg)	Sodium (mg)	Carbo (g)	Protein (g)
Condiments									
Sauce Packet	.5 oz.	15	0	0	0	0	180	4	0
BBQ Dipping Sauce	1 oz.	40	0	0	0	0	350	10	0
Au Jus Sauce	3 oz.	5	0	.05	.02	0	386	.89	.30
BBQ Vinaigrette Dressing	2 oz.	140	99	11	1.5	0	660	9	0
Bleu Cheese Dressing	2 oz.	300	279	31	6	45	580	3	2
Bronco Berry Sauce	1.5 oz.	90	0	0	0	0	35	23	0
Buttermilk Ranch Drsng.	2 oz.	360	349	39	6	5	490	2	1
Butter. Ran. Drsng. no fat	2 oz.	60	0	0	0	0	750	13	1
Caesar Dressing	2 oz.	310	310	34	5	60	470	1	1
Croutons, Cheese&Garlic	.63 oz.	100	53	6.25	n/a	n/a	138	10	2.5
Croutons, Seasoned	.25 oz.	30	10	1	0	0	70	5	1
German Mustard Packet	.25 oz.	5	0	0	0	0	60	0	0
Honey French Dressing	2 oz.	290	209	24	4	0	410	18	0
Honey Mustard Sauce	1 oz.	130	111	12	1.5	10	160	5	0
Horsey Sauce Packet	.5 oz.	60	45	5	0.5	5	150	3	0
Italian Dressing	2 oz.	25	10	1	1	0	1030	3	0
Italian Parmesan Dressing	2 oz.	240	221	24	4	0	950	4	1
Ketchup Packet	.32 oz.	10	0	0	0	0	100	2	0
French Toast Syrup	.5 oz.	130	0	0	0	0	45	32	0
Mayonnaise Packet	.44 oz.	90	90	10	1.5	10	65	0	0
Mayonnaise Packet Light	.44 oz.	20	15	1.5	0	0	110	1	0
Marinara Sauce	1.5 oz.	35	12	1	0	0	260	4	1
Tangy Southwest Sauce	1.5 oz.	250	240	26	4.5	30	290	3	0
Thousand Island Dressing	2 oz.	290	249	28	4.5	35	480	9	1
Beverages									
Milk	1	120	43	5	3	20	120	12	8
Hot Chocolate	1	110	11	1	0.5	0	120	23	2
Orange Juice	1	140	0	0	0	0	0	34	1
Vanilla Shake	1	470	141	15	7	45	360	83	10
Chocolate Shake	1	480	149	16	8	45	370	84	10
Strawberry Shake	1	500	120	13	8	15	340	87	11
Jamocha Shake	1	470	141	15	7	45	390	82	10

Burger King®

Breakfast
Croissan'wich w/Egg/Ch.	1	320	170	19	7	185	730	24	12
Croissan' w/Sau../Egg/Ch.	1	520	350	39	14	210	1090	24	19
Croissan' w/Bac./Egg/Ch.	1	360	200	22	8	195	950	25	15
Croissan' w/Ham/Egg/Ch.	1	360	180	20	8	200	1500	25	18

Food Item	Amount	Total Calories	Fat Calories	Total Fat (g)	Sat. Fat (g)	Chol. (mg)	Sodium (mg)	Carbo (g)	Protein (g)
French Toast Sticks	5	390	180	20	4.5	0	440	46	7
Hash Brown Rounds	1	230	130	15	4	0	450	23	2

Burgers

Food Item	Amount	Total Calories	Fat Calories	Total Fat (g)	Sat. Fat (g)	Chol. (mg)	Sodium (mg)	Carbo (g)	Protein (g)
Whopper	1	700	370	42	13	85	1020	52	31
Whopper w/Cheese	1	800	440	49	18	110	1450	53	35
Double Whopper	1	970	550	61	23	160	1110	52	52
Double Whop. w/Cheese	1	1060	620	69	27	185	1540	53	56
Whopper Jr.	1	390	200	22	7	45	550	31	17
Whopper Jr. w/Cheese	1	430	230	26	9	55	770	32	19
Chicken Whopper	1	570	230	25	4.5	75	1410	48	38
Hamburger	1	310	120	13	5	40	550	30	17
Cheeseburger	1	350	150	17	8	50	770	31	19
Double Hamburger	1	440	210	23	10	75	600	30	28
Double Cheeseburger	1	530	280	31	15	100	1030	32	32
Bacon Cheeseburger	1	390	180	20	9	60	990	31	22
Bacon Double Cheese.	1	770	310	34	17	110	1250	31	35
Angus Steak Burger	1	570	200	22	8	180	1270	62	33
Angus Bac./Ch./St. Burger	1	710	300	33	15	215	1990	64	41
Low Carb Ang. St. Burger	1	280	160	18	7	180	730	5	25
Low Carb B.&C. St. Bur.	1	420	270	29	14	215	1450	7	33
Veggie w/Mayo	1	380	140	16	2.5	5	930	46	14

Sandwich/Side Orders

Food Item	Amount	Total Calories	Fat Calories	Total Fat (g)	Sat. Fat (g)	Chol. (mg)	Sodium (mg)	Carbo (g)	Protein (g)
Chicken Sandwich	1	560	260	28	6	60	1270	52	25
TenderCrisp Ch. Sand.	1	780	400	45	7	55	1710	70	27
Spicy T. Cr. Ch. Sand.	1	720	340	38	6	55	2030	71	27
Fish Filet Sandwich	1	710	270	30	18	55	840	44	18
Chicken Tenders	5	210	110	12	3.5	30	530	13	14
Chicken Tenders	8	340	170	19	5	50	840	20	22
Chicken Caesar Salad	1	190	60	7	3	50	900	9	25
Shrimp Caesar Salad	1	180	90	10	3	120	800	9	19
Chicken Garden Salad	1	210	60	7	3	50	910	13	26
Shrimp Garden Salad	1	200	90	10	3	120	890	12	20
Side Garden Salad	1	20	0	0	0	0	15	4	1
French Fries (small)	1	230	100	11	3	0	410	29	3
French Fries (medium)	1	360	160	18	5	0	640	46	4
French Fries (large)	1	500	220	25	7	0	880	63	6
French Fries (king)	1	600	270	30	8	0	1070	76	7
Onion Rings (small)	1	180	80	9	2	0	260	22	3
Onion Rings (medium)	1	320	140	16	4	0	460	40	4
Onion Rings (large)	1	480	210	23	6	0	690	60	7
Onion Rings (king size)	1	550	240	27	7	0	800	70	8
Chili	1	190	70	8	3	25	1040	17	13

Food Item	Amount	Total Calories	Fat Calories	Total Fat (g)	Sat. Fat (g)	Chol. (mg)	Sodium (mg)	Carbo (g)	Protein (g)
Desserts									
Dutch Apple Pie	1	340	130	14	3	3	470	52	2
Hershey's Sundae Pie	1	310	160	18	13	10	130	35	3
Vanilla Shake (small)	1	330	50	6	4	20	260	61	9
Vanilla Shake (medium)	1	430	70	8	5	25	340	79	12
Chocolate Shake (small)	1	400	50	6	4	20	360	77	10
Chocolate Shake (med.)	1	500	70	8	5	25	440	95	13
Strawberry Shake (small)	1	390	50	6	4	20	270	76	9
Strawberry Shake (med.)	1	500	70	8	5	25	350	95	12
Nestle Toll House cookies	1	440	150	16	5	20	360	68	5

Chick-fil-A®

Food Item	Amount	Total Calories	Fat Calories	Total Fat (g)	Sat. Fat (g)	Chol. (mg)	Sodium (mg)	Carbo (g)	Protein (g)
Sandwiches									
Chicken	1	410	150	16	3.5	60	1300	38	28
Chicken Deluxe	1	420	150	16	3.5	60	1300	39	28
Chargrilled Chicken	1	270	30	3.5	1	65	940	33	28
Chargrilled Chicken Club	1	380	100	11	5	90	1240	33	35
Cool Wraps									
Chargrilled Chicken	1	390	60	7	3	65	1020	54	29
Chicken Caesar	1	460	90	10	6	80	1350	52	36
Spicy Chicken	1	380	60	6	3	60	1090	52	30
Specialties									
Chick-n-strips	1	290	120	13	2.5	65	730	14	29
Nuggets	1	260	110	12	2.5	70	1090	12	26
Chicken Salad Sandwich	1	350	140	15	3	65	880	32	20
Hearty Breast of Ch. Soup	1	140	35	3.5	1	25	900	18	8
Salads									
Chargrilled Ch. Garden	1	180	60	6	3	65	620	9	22
Southwest Char. Garden	1	240	70	8	3.5	60	770	17	25
Chick-n-strips	1	390	160	18	5	80	860	22	34
Side Items									
Side Salad	1	60	25	3	1.5	10	75	4	3
Cole Slaw	1	260	280	21	3.5	25	220	17	2
Carrot & Raisin Salad	1	170	50	6	1	10	110	28	1
Waffle Potato Fries	1	280	120	14	5	15	105	37	3
Fresh Fruit Cup	1	60	0	0	0	0	0	16	1

Food Item	Amount	Total Calories	Fat Calories	Total Fat (g)	Sat. Fat (g)	Chol. (mg)	Sodium (mg)	Carbo (g)	Protein (g)
Dipping Sauces									
Polynesian	1	110	50	6	1	0	210	13	0
Barbeque	1	45	0	0	0	0	180	11	0
Honey Mustard	1	45	0	0	0	0	150	10	0
Buttermilk Ranch	1	110	110	12	2	5	200	1	0
Buffalo	1	15	15	1.5	0	0	410	1	0
Honey Roasted BBQ	1	60	50	6	1	5	90	2	0
Croutons/Kernels									
Garlic Butter Croutons	1	50	30	3	0	0	90	6	1
Hon. Roast, Sun. Ker.	1	80	60	7	1	0	38	3	2.5
Tortilla Strips	1	70	30	3.5	.5	0	53	9	2
Dressings									
Caesar	2.5	160	150	17	2.5	30	240	1	1
Red. Fat Rasp. Vinaigrette	2	80	20	2	0	0	190	15	0
Blue Cheese	2.5	150	140	16	3	20	300	1	1
Buttermilk Ranch	2.5	160	150	16	2.5	5	270	1	0
Spicy	2.5	140	130	14	2	5	130	2	0
Thousand Island	2.5	150	130	14	2	10	250	5	0
Light Italian	2	15	5	.5	0	0	570	2	0
Fat Free Honey Mustard	2	60	0	0	0	0	200	14	0
Desserts									
Icedream Cup	1	230	50	6	3.5	25	100	38	5
Icedream Cone	1	160	35	4	2	15	80	28	4
Lemon Pie	1	320	90	10	3.5	110	220	51	7
Fudge Nut Brownie	1	330	140	15	3.5	20	210	45	4
Cheesecake	1	340	190	21	12	90	270	30	6
Breakfast Ingredients									
Plain Biscuit	1	260	90	11	2.5	0	670	38	4
Hot Buttered Biscuit	1	270	110	12	3	0	680	38	4
Chicken Biscuit	1	400	160	18	4.5	30	1200	43	16
Ch. Biscuit with Cheese	1	450	200	23	7	45	1430	43	19
Biscuit with Bacon	1	300	130	14	4	5	780	38	6
Biscuit w/Bacon and Egg	1	390	180	20	6	250	860	38	13
Bis. w/Bacon, Egg, & Ch.	1	430	220	24	9	265	1070	38	16
Biscuit with Egg	1	340	150	16	4.5	245	740	38	11
Biscuit with Egg & Ch.	1	390	190	21	7	260	960	38	13
Biscuit with Sausage	1	410	210	23	9	20	740	42	9
Biscuit with Saus. & Egg	1	500	260	29	11	265	810	43	15
Biscuit w/Saus./Egg/Ch.	1	540	300	33	13	280	1030	43	18
Biscuit with Gravy	1	310	120	13	3.5	5	930	44	5

Food Item	Amount	Total Calories	Fat Calories	Total Fat (g)	Sat. Fat (g)	Chol. (mg)	Sodium (mg)	Carbo (g)	Protein (g)
Hashbrowns	1	170	80	9	4.5	10	350	20	2
Danish	1	430	150	17	4.5	25	160	63	6

Dairy Queen®

Burgers

Homestyle Hamburger	1	290	110	12	5	45	630	29	17
Homestyle Cheeseburger	1	340	150	17	8	55	850	29	20
Home. Double Cheese.	1	540	280	31	16	115	1130	30	35
Home. Bac. Dble. Cheese.	1	610	320	36	18	130	1380	31	41
Ultimate Burger	1	670	390	43	19	135	1210	29	40

Hot Dogs

Hot Dog	1	240	120	14	5	25	730	19	9
Chili 'n' Cheese Dog	1	330	190	21	9	45	1090	22	14

Sandwiches/Baskets

Breaded Chicken Sand.	1	510	240	27	4	40	1070	47	19
Grilled Chick. Sandwich	1	340	150	16	2.5	50	1000	26	22
Chicken Strip Basket	1	1000	450	50	13	55	2510	102	35

Fries/Onion Rings

French Fries (small)	1	300	110	12	2.5	0	700	45	3
French Fries (medium)	1	380	140	15	3	0	880	56	4
French Fries (large)	1	480	170	19	4	0	1140	72	5
Onion Rings	1	470	270	30	6	0	740	45	6

Salads

Crispy Chicken (no dress.)	1	350	180	20	6	40	620	21	21
Grilled Chick. (no dress.)	1	240	90	10	5	65	950	12	26
Side Salad	1	60	25	2.5	1.5	5	60	6	3

Salad Dressings

Honey Mustard	1	260	190	21	3.5	20	370	18	1
Wish-bone Fat Free Ital.	1	25	0	0	0	0	520	6	0
Blue Cheese	1	210	180	20	4	5	700	4	2
Ranch	1	310	300	33	5	25	390	3	1
Fat Free Honey Mustard	1	50	0	0	0	0	160	13	0
Red. Cal. Buttermilk	1	140	120	13	2	15	390	5	0
Fat Free Thousand Island	1	60	0	0	0	0	400	16	0
Fat Free Ranch	1	60	0	0	0	0	410	13	1
Fat Free Red French	1	40	0	0	0	0	330	10	0
Fat Free Italian	1	10	0	0	0	0	390	3	0
Fat Free Buttermilk Ran.	1	30	0	0	0	0	440	6	1

Food Item	Amount	Total Calories	Fat Calories	Total Fat (g)	Sat. Fat (g)	Chol. (mg)	Sodium (mg)	Carbo (g)	Protein (g)
Cones									
Vanilla Soft Serve	1/2 cup	140	40	4.5	3	15	70	22	3
Chocolate Soft Serve	1/2 cup	150	45	5	3.5	15	75	22	4
Small Vanilla	1	230	60	7	4.5	20	115	38	6
Medium Vanilla	1	330	90	9	6	30	160	53	8
Large Vanilla	1	480	130	15	9	45	230	76	11
Small Chocolate	1	240	70	8	5	20	115	37	6
Medium Chocolate	1	340	100	11	7	30	160	53	8
Small Dipped	1	340	150	17	9	20	130	42	6
Medium Dipped	1	490	220	24	13	30	190	59	8
Large Dipped	1	710	330	36	17	45	250	85	12
Malts, Shakes, and Misty									
Small Choc. Malt	1	640	150	16	11	55	340	111	15
Medium Choc. Malt	1	870	200	22	14	70	450	153	20
Large Choc. Malt	1	1320	310	35	22	110	670	222	29
Small Choc. Shake	1	560	140	15	10	50	280	93	13
Medium Choc. Shake	1	760	180	20	12	70	370	129	17
Large Choc. Shake	1	1140	300	33	21	105	550	186	26
Small Misty Slush	1	220	0	0	0	0	20	56	0
Medium Misty Slush	1	290	0	0	0	0	30	74	0
Sundaes									
Small Strawberry	1	240	60	7	4.5	20	110	40	5
Medium Strawberry	1	340	80	9	6	30	160	58	7
Large Strawberry	1	500	130	15	9	45	230	83	10
Small Chocolate	1	280	60	7	4.5	20	140	49	5
Medium Chocolate	1	400	90	10	6	30	210	71	8
Large Chocolate	1	580	140	15	10	45	260	100	11
Royal Treats									
Banana Split	1	510	100	12	8	30	180	96	8
Peanut Buster Parfait	1	730	280	31	17	35	400	99	16
Pecan Praline Parfait	1	720	260	29	11	30	610	105	9
Triple Chocolate Utopia	1	770	350	39	17	55	390	96	12
Strawberry Shortcake	1	430	120	14	9	60	360	70	7
Brownie Earthquake	1	740	240	27	16	50	350	112	10
Novelties									
DQ Sandwich	1	220	60	6	3	10	140	31	4
Chocolate Dilly Bar	1	210	120	13	7	10	75	21	3
Buster Bar	1	450	260	28	12	15	280	41	10
Starkiss	1	80	0	0	0	0	10	21	0
Fudge Bar	1	50	0	0	0	0	70	13	4

Food Item	Amount	Total Calories	Fat Calories	Total Fat (g)	Sat. Fat (g)	Chol. (mg)	Sodium (mg)	Carbo (g)	Protein (g)
Vanilla Orange Bar	1	60	0	0	0	0	40	17	2
Lemon DQ Freez'r	1/2 cup	80	0	0	0	0	10	20	0

Blizzard Treats

Food Item	Amount	Total Calories	Fat Calories	Total Fat (g)	Sat. Fat (g)	Chol. (mg)	Sodium (mg)	Carbo (g)	Protein (g)
Small Oreo Cookies	1	570	190	21	10	40	430	83	11
Medium Oreo Cookies	1	700	240	26	12	45	560	103	13
Large Oreo Cookies	1	1010	340	37	18	70	770	148	19
Small Choc. Chip Ck. D.	1	720	250	28	14	50	370	105	12
Med. Choc. Chip Ck. D.	1	1030	360	40	20	70	520	150	17
Large Choc. Chip Ck. D.	1	1320	470	52	26	90	670	193	21
Small Banana Split	1	460	130	14	9	40	210	73	10
Medium Banana Split	1	580	150	17	11	50	260	97	12
Large Banana Split	1	810	210	23	15	70	360	134	17

Domino's Pizza®

12" Cheese

Food Item	Amount	Total Calories	Fat Calories	Total Fat (g)	Sat. Fat (g)	Chol. (mg)	Sodium (mg)	Carbo (g)	Protein (g)
Hand-Tossed	1/8	186	-	5.5	2	9	385	28	7
Deep Dish	1/8	238	-	11	3.5	11	555	28	9
Crunch Thin	1/8	137	-	7	2.5	10	292	14	5

12" Pepperoni

Food Item	Amount	Total Calories	Fat Calories	Total Fat (g)	Sat. Fat (g)	Chol. (mg)	Sodium (mg)	Carbo (g)	Protein (g)
Hand-Tossed	1/8	223	-	9	3.5	16	521	28	9
Deep Dish	1/8	275	-	14	5	19	692	14	5
Crunch Thin	1/8	174	-	10	4	17	429	14	7

12" Sausage

Food Item	Amount	Total Calories	Fat Calories	Total Fat (g)	Sat. Fat (g)	Chol. (mg)	Sodium (mg)	Carbo (g)	Protein (g)
Hand-Tossed	1/8	231	-	9.5	3.5	17	530	28	9
Deep Dish	1/8	283	-	15	5	19	701	29	11
Crunch Thin	1/8	206	-	13.5	5	23	533	14	8

12" Pepperoni & Sausage

Food Item	Amount	Total Calories	Fat Calories	Total Fat (g)	Sat. Fat (g)	Chol. (mg)	Sodium (mg)	Carbo (g)	Protein (g)
Hand-Tossed	1/8	255	-	11.5	4.5	22	625	28	10
Deep Dish	1/8	307	-	17	6	25	796	29	12
Crunch Thin	1/8	206	-	13.5	5	23	533	14	8

12" Ham & Pineapple

Food Item	Amount	Total Calories	Fat Calories	Total Fat (g)	Sat. Fat (g)	Chol. (mg)	Sodium (mg)	Carbo (g)	Protein (g)
Hand-Tossed	1/8	200	-	6	2.5	12	466	29	9
Deep Dish	1/8	252	-	1.5	4	15	637	30	10
Crunch Thin	1/8	150	-	7.5	3	13	374	15	7

12" Ham

Food Item	Amount	Total Calories	Fat Calories	Total Fat (g)	Sat. Fat (g)	Chol. (mg)	Sodium (mg)	Carbo (g)	Protein (g)
Hand-Tossed	1/8	198	-	6	2.5	13	492	28	9
Deep Dish	1/8	250	-	11.5	4	16	663	28	11
Crunch Thin	1/8	148	-	7.5	3	14	399	14	7

12" Green Pepper, Onion, & Mushroom

Food Item	Amount	Total Calories	Fat Calories	Total Fat (g)	Sat. Fat (g)	Chol. (mg)	Sodium (mg)	Carbo (g)	Protein (g)
Hand-Tossed	1/8	191	-	5.5	2	9	385	29	8

Food Item	Amount	Total Calories	Fat Calories	Total Fat (g)	Sat. Fat (g)	Chol. (mg)	Sodium (mg)	Carbo (g)	Protein (g)
Deep Dish	1/8	244	-	11	3.5	11	556	30	9
Crunch Thin	1/8	142	-	7.5	2.5	10	293	15	6
12" Beef									
Hand-Tossed	1/8	225	-	9	3.5	16	493	28	9
Deep Dish	1/8	277	-	14.5	5	19	663	28	11
Crunch Thin	1/8	175	-	10.5	4	17	400	14	7
Side Dishes									
Buffalo Chicken Kickers	1	47	-	2	.5	9	162	3	4
Hot Buffalo Wings	1	45	-	2.5	.5	26	254	3	5
BBQ Buffalo Wings	1	50	-	2.5	.5	26	175	2	6
Hot Dipping Sauce	1	15	-	0	0	0	1820	4	0
Blue Cheese Dipping Sauce	1	223	-	23.5	4	20	417	2	1
Ranch Dipping Sauce	1	197	-	20.5	3	9	380	2	1
Breadsticks	1	115	-	6.3	1.1	0	122	12	2
Cheesy Bread	1	123	-	6.5	1.9	6	162	13	4
Marinara Dipping Sauce	1	25	-	.2	0	0	262	5	1
Garlic Sauce	1	440	-	49	10	0	380	0	0
Cinna Stix	1	123	-	6	1	0	111	15	2
Sweet Icing	1	250	-	2.5	2.5	0	0	57	0

Kentucky Fried Chicken®

Chicken

Food Item	Amount	Total Calories	Fat Calories	Total Fat (g)	Sat. Fat (g)	Chol. (mg)	Sodium (mg)	Carbo (g)	Protein (g)
Original Recipe									
Whole Wing	1	150	90	9	2.5	60	370	5	11
Chicken Breast	1	380	220	19	6	145	1150	11	40
Drumstick	1	140	80	8	2	75	440	4	4
Thigh	1	360	160	25	7	165	1060	12	22
Extra Crispy									
Whole Wing	1	180	140	12	4	55	390	10	10
Breast	1	460	240	28	8	160	874	17	39
Drumstick	1	160	110	10	2.5	70	420	5	12
Thigh	1	370	250	26	7	120	710	12	21
Hot & Spicy									
Whole Wing	1	180	130	11	8	60	420	9	11
Breast	1	460	270	27	8	130	1450	20	33
Drumstick	1	150	90	9	2.5	65	380	4	13
Thigh	1	400	225	28	8	125	1240	14	22

Food Item	Amount	Total Calories	Fat Calories	Total Fat (g)	Sat. Fat (g)	Chol. (mg)	Sodium (mg)	Carbo (g)	Protein (g)
Sandwiches									
Original Recipe									
w/Sauce	1	450	240	27	6	65	1010	22	29
no sauce	1	320	120	13	4	60	890	21	29
Triple Crunch									
w/Sauce	1	670	360	40	8	80	1640	42	36
no sauce	1	540	230	26	6	75	1510	41	35
Triple Crunch Zinger									
w/Sauce	1	680	370	41	8	90	1650	42	35
no sauce	1	540	230	26	6	75	1510	41	35
Tender Roast									
w/Sauce	1	390	170	19	4	70	810	24	31
no sauce	1	260	45	5	1.5	65	690	23	31
Honey BBQ Flavored	1	300	50	6	1.5	150	640	41	21
Twister	1	670	300	38	7	60	1650	55	27
Crispy Strips									
Colonel's Crispy Strips	3	400	125	24	5	75	1250	17	29
Popcorn Chicken									
Small	1	450	270	29	6	50	1030	26	19
Large	1	650	400	43	10	70	1530	38	29
Pot Pie									
Chunky Chicken	1	770	378	40	15	115	1680	70	33
Wings									
Hot Wings Pieces	6	450	297	29	6	145	1120	23	24
Honey BBQ Wings	6	540	300	33	7	-	1130	36	15
Vegetables									
Mashed Potatoes w/Gravy	1	120	40	4.5	1	0	380	18	2
Potato Wedges	1	240	110	12	3	0	830	30	5
Macaroni & Cheese	1	130	50	6	2	5	610	15	5
Corn on the Cob	1	150	25	3	1	0	10	26	5
BBQ Baked Beans	1	230	10	1	1	0	720	46	8
Cole Slaw	1	190	100	11	2	5	300	22	1
Potato Salad	1	150	80	9	1.5	5	470	22	2
Green Beans	1	50	10	1.5	0	5	570	7	2
Breads									
Biscuit	1	190	90	10	2	1.5	580	23	2
Desserts									
Chocolate Chip Cake	1	320	140	16	4	55	230	41	4

Food Item	Amount	Total Calories	Fat Calories	Total Fat (g)	Sat. Fat (g)	Chol. (mg)	Sodium (mg)	Carbo (g)	Protein (g)
Fudge Brownie Parfait	1	280	90	10	3.5	145	190	44	3
Lemon Creme Parfait	1	410	130	14	8	20	290	62	7
Chocolate Creme Parfait	1	290	130	15	11	15	330	37	3
Straw. Shortcake Parfait	1	200	60	7	6	10	220	33	1
Pecan Pie Slice	1	490	200	23	5	65	510	66	5
Apple Pie Slice	1	310	130	14	3	0	280	44	2
Straw. Creme Pie Slice	1	280	130	15	8	15	130	32	4

McDonald's®

Sandwiches

Hamburger	1	280	90	10	4	30	550	36	12
Cheeseburger	1	330	130	14	6	45	790	36	15
Double Cheeseburger	1	490	240	26	12	85	1220	38	25
Quarter Pounder	1	430	190	21	8	70	770	38	23
Quar. Pounder w/Cheese	1	540	260	29	13	95	1240	39	29
D. Quar. Pound. w/Cheese	1	770	430	47	20	165	1440	39	46
Big Mac	1	600	300	33	11	85	1050	50	8
Big N' Tasty	1	540	290	32	10	80	780	38	9
Big N' Tasty w/Cheese	1	590	330	36	12	95	1020	39	9
Filet-O-Fish	1	410	180	20	4	45	660	41	15
Chicken McGrill	1	400	140	16	3	70	1020	37	27
Crispy Chicken	1	510	230	26	4.5	50	1090	47	22
McChicken®	1	430	200	23	4.5	45	830	41	14
Hot 'n Spicy McChicken	1	450	230	26	5	45	820	40	15

French Fries

Small	1	220	100	11	2	0	150	28	3
Medium	1	350	150	17	3	0	220	44	5
Large	1	520	230	25	4.5	0	340	66	7
Ketchup Packet	1	10	0	0	0	0	115	3	0
Salt Packet	1	0	0	0	0	0	270	0	0

Chicken McNuggets

Chicken McNuggets	4	170	90	10	2	25	450	10	10
Chicken McNuggets	6	250	130	15	3	35	670	15	15
Chicken McNuggets	10	420	220	24	5	60	1120	26	25
Chicken McNuggets	20	840	440	49	11	125	2240	51	50
Barbeque Sauce	1	45	0	0	0	0	250	10	0
Honey	1	45	0	0	0	0	0	12	0
Hot Mustard Sauce	1	60	30	3.5	0	5	240	7	1
Sweet 'N Sour Sauce	1	50	0	0	0	0	140	11	0

Food Item	Amount	Total Calories	Fat Calories	Total Fat (g)	Sat. Fat (g)	Chol. (mg)	Sodium (mg)	Carbo (g)	Protein (g)
Chicken Selects Premium Breast Strips									
Premium Breast Strips	3	380	170	19	3	50	960	28	23
Premium Breast Strips	5	630	290	32	5	85	1590	47	38
Premium Breast Strips	10	1250	570	64	10	170	3180	94	76
Spicy Buffalo Sauce	1	60	60	7	1	0	430	2	0
Creamy Ranch Sauce	1	210	200	22	3.5	10	310	2	0
Tangy Honey Mustard Sauce	1	70	25	2.5	0	10	170	12	1
Salads									
Gr. Chick./Bacon/Ranch	1	250	90	10	4.5	85	930	9	31
Cr. Chick./Bacon Ranch	1	350	180	19	6	65	1000	20	26
Bacon Ranch	1	130	70	8	4	25	280	7	10
Grilled Chicken Caesar	1	200	50	6	3	70	820	9	29
Crispy Chicken Caesar	1	310	140	16	4.5	50	890	20	23
Caesar	1	90	35	4	2.5	10	170	7	7
Gr. Ch. California Cobb	1	270	100	11	5	145	1060	9	33
Cr. Ch. California Cobb	1	370	190	21	6	125	1130	20	27
California Cobb w/o Ch.	1	150	80	9	4.5	85	410	7	11
Side	1	15	0	0	0	0	10	3	1
Butter Garlic Croutons	1	50	15	1.5	0	0	140	8	1
Fiesta w/Sour Cr./Salsa	1	450	250	27	13	95	920	28	24
Fiesta with Salsa	1	390	200	22	10	80	870	26	23
Fiesta with Sour Cream	1	420	240	27	13	95	630	21	22
Fiesta	1	360	200	22	10	80	580	19	21
Salad Dressings									
Newman's Own Cobb	2 F oz.	120	80	9	1.5	10	440	9	1
New. Own Cr. Caesar	2 F oz.	190	170	18	3.5	20	500	4	2
N. O. Low Fat Bal. Vin.	1.5 F oz.	40	25	3	0	0	730	4	0
Newman's Own Ranch	2 F oz.	170	130	15	2.5	20	530	9	1
Newman's Own Salsa	3 F oz.	30	0	0	0	0	290	7	1
Breakfast									
Egg McMuffin	1	300	110	12	5	235	850	28	18
Sausage McMuffin	1	370	200	23	9	50	790	28	14
Sausage McMuffin w/Egg	1	450	250	28	10	260	940	29	20
English Muffin	1	150	15	2	0.5	0	260	27	5
Bacon/Egg/Cheese Bis.	1	430	230	26	8	240	1230	31	18
Sausage Biscuit with Egg	1	490	300	33	10	245	1010	31	16
Sausage Biscuit	1	410	250	28	8	35	930	30	10
Biscuit	1	240	100	11	2.5	0	640	30	4
McGriddles									
Bacon/Egg/Ch.	1	440	190	21	7	240	1270	43	19

Food Item	Amount	Total Calories	Fat Calories	Total Fat (g)	Sat. Fat (g)	Chol. (mg)	Sodium (mg)	Carbo (g)	Protein (g)
Saus./Egg/Ch.	1	550	300	33	11	260	1290	43	20
Sausage	1	420	210	23	7	35	970	42	11
Ham/Egg/Cheese Bagel	1	550	200	23	8	255	1500	58	26
Spanish Omelet Bagel	1	710	360	40	15	275	1520	59	27
Steak/Egg/Cheese Bagel	1	640	280	31	12	265	1540	57	31
Bagel (plain)	1	260	10	1	0	0	520	54	9
Big Breakfast	1	700	420	47	13	455	1430	45	24
Deluxe Breakfast	1	1190	550	61	15	470	1990	130	30
Sausage Burrito	1	290	150	16	6	170	680	24	13
Hotcakes and Sausage	1	780	300	33	9	50	1060	104	15
Hotcakes (marg. & syrup)	1	600	150	17	3	20	770	104	9
Sausage	1	170	150	16	5	35	290	0	6
Scrambled Eggs	2	160	100	11	3.5	425	170	1	13
Hash Browns	1	130	70	8	1.5	0	330	14	1
Warm Cinnamon Roll	1	440	170	19	5	80	330	60	7
Del. Warm Cin. Roll	1	510	210	23	8	60	660	81	8
Grape Jam	.5 oz.	35	0	0	0	0	0	9	0
Strawberry Preserves	.5 oz.	35	0	0	0	0	0	9	0

Desserts/Shakes

Food Item	Amount	Total Calories	Fat Calories	Total Fat (g)	Sat. Fat (g)	Chol. (mg)	Sodium (mg)	Carbo (g)	Protein (g)
Fruit 'n Yogurt Parfait	1	160	20	2	1	5	85	30	4
F. 'n Y. Par. w/o granola	1	130	15	2	1	5	55	25	4
Apple Dippers	1	35	0	0	0	0	0	8	0
Ap. Dip. w/Low Fat Car.	1	100	5	1	0.5	5	35	22	0
Low Fat Caramel Dip	.8 oz.	70	5	1	0.5	5	35	14	0
Van. Rd. Fat Ice Cr. Cone	1	150	40	4.5	3	20	75	23	4
Kiddie Cone	1	45	15	1.5	1	5	20	7	1
Strawberry Sundae	1	290	70	7	5	30	95	50	7
Hot Caramel Sundae	1	360	90	10	6	35	180	61	7
Hot Fudge Sundae	1	340	100	12	9	30	170	52	8
Nuts (for Sundaes)	.3 oz.	40	30	3.5	0	0	55	2	2
M&M McFlurry	1	630	200	23	15	75	210	90	16
Oreo McFlurry	1	570	180	20	12	70	280	82	15
Choc. Triple Thick Shake	12 F oz.	430	110	12	8	50	210	70	11
Choc. Triple Thick Shake	16 F oz.	580	150	17	11	65	280	94	15
Choc. Triple Thick Shake	21 F oz.	750	200	22	14	90	360	123	19
Choc. Triple Thick Shake	32 F oz.	1150	300	33	22	135	550	187	30
Straw. Triple Thick Shake	12 F oz.	420	110	12	8	50	140	67	11
Straw. Triple Thick Shake	16 F oz.	560	150	16	11	65	190	89	14
Straw. Triple Thick Shake	21 F oz.	730	190	21	14	90	250	116	19
Straw. Triple Thick Shake	32 F oz.	1120	290	32	22	135	380	178	28
Van. Triple Thick Shake	12 F oz.	430	110	12	8	50	300	67	11
Van. Triple Thick Shake	16 F oz.	570	150	16	11	65	400	89	14

Food Item	Amount	Total Calories	Fat Calories	Total Fat (g)	Sat. Fat (g)	Chol. (mg)	Sodium (mg)	Carbo (g)	Protein (g)
Van. Triple Thick Shake	21 F oz.	750	190	21	14	90	530	116	18
Van. Triple Thick Shake	32 F oz.	1140	290	32	22	135	810	178	28
Baked Apple Pie	1	260	120	13	3.5	0	200	34	3
Mc. Choc. Chip Cookies	2 oz.	280	130	14	8	40	170	37	3
Mc. Cookies	2 oz.	230	70	8	2	0	250	38	3
Chocolate Chip Cookie	1	160	70	8	2	5	125	22	2
Oatmeal Raisin Cookie	1	150	50	6	1	5	100	23	2
Sugar Cookie	1	140	60	6	1	10	120	20	2

Pizza Hut®

12" Medium Pan Pizza

Food Item	Amount	Total Calories	Fat Calories	Total Fat (g)	Sat. Fat (g)	Chol. (mg)	Sodium (mg)	Carbo (g)	Protein (g)
Cheese Only	1 piece	280	120	13	5	25	500	29	11
Pepperoni	1 piece	290	130	15	5	25	560	29	11
Quartered Ham	1 piece	260	100	11	4	20	540	29	11
Supreme	1 piece	320	150	16	6	25	650	30	13
Super Supreme	1 piece	340	160	18	6	35	760	30	14
Chicken Supreme	1 piece	280	100	12	4	25	530	30	13
Meat Lover's	1 piece	340	170	19	7	35	750	29	15
Veggie Lover's	1 piece	260	100	12	4	15	470	30	10
Pepperoni Lover's	1 piece	340	170	19	7	40	700	29	15
Sausage Lover's	1 piece	330	160	17	6	30	640	29	13

12" Medium Thin 'N Crispy Pizza

Food Item	Amount	Total Calories	Fat Calories	Total Fat (g)	Sat. Fat (g)	Chol. (mg)	Sodium (mg)	Carbo (g)	Protein (g)
Cheese Only	1 piece	200	80	8	4.5	25	490	21	10
Pepperoni	1 piece	210	90	10	4.5	25	550	21	10
Quartered Ham	1 piece	180	60	6	3	20	530	21	10
Supreme	1 piece	240	100	11	5	25	640	22	11
Super Supreme	1 piece	260	120	13	6	35	760	23	13
Chicken Supreme	1 piece	200	60	7	3.5	25	520	22	12
Meat Lover's	1 piece	270	130	14	6	35	740	21	13
Veggie Lover's	1 piece	180	60	7	3	15	480	23	8
Pepperoni Lover's	1 piece	260	120	14	7	40	690	21	13
Sausage Lover's	1 piece	240	110	13	6	30	630	21	11

12" Medium Hand-Tossed Pizza

Food Item	Amount	Total Calories	Fat Calories	Total Fat (g)	Sat. Fat (g)	Chol. (mg)	Sodium (mg)	Carbo (g)	Protein (g)
Cheese Only	1 piece	240	70	8	4.5	25	520	30	12
Pepperoni	1 piece	250	80	9	4.5	25	570	29	12
Quartered Ham	1 piece	220	50	6	3	20	550	29	12
Supreme	1 piece	270	100	11	5	25	660	30	12
Super Supreme	1 piece	300	110	13	6	35	780	31	15
Chicken Supreme	1 piece	230	60	6	3	25	550	30	14
Meat Lover's	1 piece	300	120	13	6	35	760	29	15

Food Item	Amount	Total Calories	Fat Calories	Total Fat (g)	Sat. Fat (g)	Chol. (mg)	Sodium (mg)	Carbo (g)	Protein (g)
Veggie Lover's	1 piece	220	60	6	3	15	490	31	10
Pepperoni Lover's	1 piece	300	120	13	7	40	710	30	15
Sausage Lover's	1 piece	280	110	12	5	30	650	30	13

14" Stuffed Crust Pizza

Food Item	Amount	Total Calories	Fat Calories	Total Fat (g)	Sat. Fat (g)	Chol. (mg)	Sodium (mg)	Carbo (g)	Protein (g)
Cheese Only	1 piece	360	120	13	8	40	920	43	18
Pepperoni	1 piece	370	130	15	8	45	970	42	18
Quartered Ham	1 piece	340	100	11	6	40	960	42	18
Supreme	1 piece	400	150	16	8	45	1070	44	20
Super Supreme	1 piece	440	180	20	9	50	1270	45	21
Chicken Supreme	1 piece	380	120	13	7	40	1020	44	20
Meat Lover's	1 piece	450	190	21	10	55	1120	43	21
Veggie Lover's	1 piece	360	120	14	7	335	980	45	16
Pepperoni Lover's	1 piece	420	170	19	10	55	1120	43	21
Sausage Lover's	1 piece	430	170	13	9	50	1130	43	19

16" Extra Large Pizza

Food Item	Amount	Total Calories	Fat Calories	Total Fat (g)	Sat. Fat (g)	Chol. (mg)	Sodium (mg)	Carbo (g)	Protein (g)
Cheese Only	1 piece	420	140	15	8	45	1080	51	20
Pepperoni	1 piece	430	150	17	8	45	1130	50	19
Quartered Ham	1 piece	380	100	12	6	45	1110	50	19
Supreme	1 piece	460	170	19	9	45	1250	53	22
Super Supreme	1 piece	490	190	21	9	55	1430	53	23
Chicken Supreme	1 piece	400	110	12	6	40	1070	52	22
Meat Lover's	1 piece	500	200	22	10	60	1400	51	24
Veggie Lover's	1 piece	390	110	12	6	30	1030	53	17
Pepperoni Lover's	1 piece	520	210	24	11	65	1370	51	25
Sausage Lover's	1 piece	510	210	23	10	55	1330	51	23

6" Personal Pan Pizza

Food Item	Amount	Total Calories	Fat Calories	Total Fat (g)	Sat. Fat (g)	Chol. (mg)	Sodium (mg)	Carbo (g)	Protein (g)
Cheese Only	1 piece	160	60	7	3	15	310	18	7
Pepperoni	1 piece	170	70	8	3	15	340	18	7
Quartered Ham	1 piece	150	50	6	2	15	330	18	7
Supreme	1 piece	190	80	9	3.5	20	420	19	8
Super Supreme	1 piece	200	90	10	4	20	480	19	9
Chicken Supreme	1 piece	160	50	6	2.5	15	320	19	8
Meat Lover's	1 piece	200	90	10	4	20	470	18	9
Veggie Lover's	1 piece	150	50	6	2	10	280	19	6
Pepperoni Lover's	1 piece	200	90	10	4.5	25	440	18	9
Sausage Lover's	1 piece	190	90	10	4	20	400	18	8

Fit 'N Delicious 12" Medium

Food Item	Amount	Total Calories	Fat Calories	Total Fat (g)	Sat. Fat (g)	Chol. (mg)	Sodium (mg)	Carbo (g)	Protein (g)
Diced Ch./R. On./Gr. Pep.	1 piece	170	40	4.5	2	15	460	23	10
Diced Ch./Mush./Jalapeno	1 piece	170	45	5	2	15	690	22	10
Ham/Red Onion/Mush.	1 piece	160	40	4.5	2	15	470	24	8

Food Item	Amount	Total Calories	Fat Calories	Total Fat (g)	Sat. Fat (g)	Chol. (mg)	Sodium (mg)	Carbo (g)	Protein (g)
Ham/Pine./D. Red Tomato	1 piece	160	35	4	2	15	470	24	8
Gr.Pep./R. On./D. R. Tom.	1 piece	150	35	4	2	15	470	24	6
Tom./Mushroom/Jalapeno	1 piece	150	40	4	2	10	590	22	6

P'Zone

Food Item	Amount	Total Calories	Fat Calories	Total Fat (g)	Sat. Fat (g)	Chol. (mg)	Sodium (mg)	Carbo (g)	Protein (g)
Pepperoni	1	610	200	22	11	55	1280	69	34
Classic	1	610	190	21	11	50	1210	71	33
Meat Lover's	1	680	250	28	14	65	1540	70	38
Marinara Dippling Sauce	1	45	0	0	0	0	380	9	2

Appetizers

Food Item	Amount	Total Calories	Fat Calories	Total Fat (g)	Sat. Fat (g)	Chol. (mg)	Sodium (mg)	Carbo (g)	Protein (g)
Hot Wings	2	110	60	6	2	70	450	1	11
Mild Wings	2	110	60	7	2	70	320	1	11
Wing Ranch Dip. Sauce	1.5 oz.	210	200	22	3.5	10	340	4	1
Wing Blue Cheese D. S.	1.5 oz.	230	210	24	5	25	550	2	2
Breadsticks	1	150	60	6	1	0	220	20	4
Cheese Breadsticks	1	200	90	10	3.5	15	340	21	7
Breadstick Dip. Sauce	3 oz.	50	0	0	0	0	370	11	1

Desserts

Food Item	Amount	Total Calories	Fat Calories	Total Fat (g)	Sat. Fat (g)	Chol. (mg)	Sodium (mg)	Carbo (g)	Protein (g)
Cinnamon Sticks	2	170	45	5	1	0	170	27	4
White Icing Dipping Cup	2 oz.	190	0	0	0	0	0	46	0
Apple Dessert Pizza	1	260	30	3.5	.5	0	250	53	4
Cherry Dessert Pizza	1	240	30	3.5	.5	0	250	47	4

Subway®

6" Sandwiches with 6 grams of fat or less

Food Item	Amount	Total Calories	Fat Calories	Total Fat (g)	Sat. Fat (g)	Chol. (mg)	Sodium (mg)	Carbo (g)	Protein (g)
Ham	1	290	45	5	1.5	25	1270	46	18
Honey Mustard Ham	1	310	45	5	2	25	1410	54	19
Oven Roasted Ch. Br.	1	236	330	50	2	45	1010	47	24
Roast Beef	1	290	45	5	2	20	910	45	19
Savory Turkey Breast	1	280	40	4	2	20	1010	46	18
Sav. Turkey Br. & Ham	1	290	45	5	2	25	1220	47	20
Sweet Onion Ch. Teriyaki	1	370	45	5	2	50	1100	58	26
Tur. Br./Ham/Roast Beef	1	320	50	6	2	35	1300	47	24
Veggie Delite	1	230	25	3	1	0	510	44	9

Breakfast Sandwiches

Food Item	Amount	Total Calories	Fat Calories	Total Fat (g)	Sat. Fat (g)	Chol. (mg)	Sodium (mg)	Carbo (g)	Protein (g)
Bacon & Egg	1	320	140	15	4	185	520	34	15
Cheese & Egg	1	320	140	15	5	185	550	34	14
Ham & Egg	1	310	110	13	4	190	720	35	16
Steak & Egg	1	330	120	14	4	190	570	35	19
Western Egg	1	300	110	12	4	180	530	36	14

Food Item	Amount	Total Calories	Fat Calories	Total Fat (g)	Sat. Fat (g)	Chol. (mg)	Sodium (mg)	Carbo (g)	Protein (g)
6" Cold Sandwiches									
BMT	1	450	190	21	8	55	1790	47	23
Cold Cut Combo	1	410	160	17	7	55	1570	46	21
Seafood Sensation	1	380	120	13	4	25	1170	52	16
Tuna	1	430	170	19	5	45	1070	46	20
Deli Style Sandwiches									
Ham	1	210	35	4	2	10	770	35	11
Roast Beef	1	220	40	4	2	15	660	35	13
Savory Turkey Breast	1	210	35	4	2	15	730	36	13
Tuna	1	300	110	13	4	25	770	36	13
6" Hot Sandwiches									
Cheese Steak	1	360	90	10	4	35	1090	47	24
Chiptole SW Ch. Steak	1	440	170	18	6	45	1160	49	24
D. Tur. Br./Ham/Bac. M.	1	470	190	21	7	55	1620	48	26
Meatball	1	500	200	22	11	45	1180	52	23
Tur. Br./Ham/Bacon Melt	1	380	110	12	5	45	1610	47	25
Classic Club	1	390	190	21	10	0	1820	13	37
Atkins Friendly Wraps									
Chicken Bacon Ranch	1	440	230	26	9	90	1550	17	43
Mediterranean Chicken	1	350	160	18	5	60	1490	17	36
Turkey Bacon Melt	1	430	240	27	10	65	1870	20	34
Turkey Breast & Ham	1	390	210	23	8	60	1890	19	32
Atkins Friendly Salads									
Classic Club w/Kr. Ranch	1	590	380	43	14	220	2370	14	38
Gr. Ch. & Baby Spinach	1	620	440	48	13	215	1480	11	39
Salads									
Garden Fresh Salad									
w/BMT meats	1	290	170	19	7	55	1360	14	17
w/Cold Cuts	1	240	140	15	6	55	1140	14	15
w/Seafood Sens.	1	210	100	11	4	25	740	20	10
w/Tuna	1	260	150	17	4	45	640	14	14
Gr. Ch. & Baby Spinach	1	420	240	26	10	0	970	10	38
Mediterranean Chicken	1	170	40	4	2	55	520	11	22
6 grams of fat or less Salads (values do not include salad dressing or croutons)									
Garden Fresh	1	60	10	1	0	0	80	11	3
GF w/Chicken	1	160	30	4	0	45	580	14	17
GF w/Ham	1	120	25	3	0	25	840	14	12
GF w/Roast Beef	1	130	30	3	1	20	480	12	13

Food Item	Amount	Total Calories	Fat Calories	Total Fat (g)	Sat. Fat (g)	Chol. (mg)	Sodium (mg)	Carbo (g)	Protein (g)
GF w/Turkey Breast	1	110	20	2	0	20	580	13	12
GF w/Tur. Breast & Ham	1	130	25	3	0	25	800	14	14
GF w/Tur./Ham/R. Beef	1	160	35	4	1	35	870	14	18

Salad Dressings

Food Item	Amount	Total Calories	Fat Calories	Total Fat (g)	Sat. Fat (g)	Chol. (mg)	Sodium (mg)	Carbo (g)	Protein (g)
Atkins Sweet as Honey M.	2 oz.	200	200	22	3	0	510	1	1
Fat Free Italian	2 oz.	35	0	0	0	0	720	7	1
Greek Vinaigrette	2 oz.	200	190	21	3	0	590	3	1
Ranch	2 oz.	200	200	22	4	10	550	1	1
Red Wine Vinaigrette	2 oz.	80	10	1	0	0	910	17	1

Salad Fixings

Food Item	Amount	Total Calories	Fat Calories	Total Fat (g)	Sat. Fat (g)	Chol. (mg)	Sodium (mg)	Carbo (g)	Protein (g)
Bacon Bits	1	60	40	4	2	20	260	0	5
Croutons	1	70	30	3	0	0	200	8	1
Diced Egg	1	45	30	3	1	120	35	0	4
Garlic Almonds	1	80	70	7	0	0	65	3	3

Cookies

Food Item	Amount	Total Calories	Fat Calories	Total Fat (g)	Sat. Fat (g)	Chol. (mg)	Sodium (mg)	Carbo (g)	Protein (g)
Chocolate Chip	1	210	90	10	4	15	160	30	2
Chocolate Chunk	1	220	90	10	4	10	105	30	2
Double Chocolate	1	210	90	10	4	15	170	30	2
M & M	1	210	90	10	4	15	105	30	2
Oatmeal Raisin	1	200	70	8	2	15	170	30	3
Peanut Butter	1	220	110	12	4	10	200	26	4
Sugar	1	230	110	12	4	15	135	28	2
White Macadamia Nut	1	220	100	11	4	15	160	28	2

Fruizie Express (small)

Food Item	Amount	Total Calories	Fat Calories	Total Fat (g)	Sat. Fat (g)	Chol. (mg)	Sodium (mg)	Carbo (g)	Protein (g)
Berry Lishus	1	110	0	0	0	0	30	28	1
Berry Lishus (w/Banana)	1	140	0	0	0	0	30	35	1
Peach Pizazz	1	100	0	0	0	0	25	26	0
Pineapple Delight	1	130	0	0	0	0	25	33	1
Pine. Delight (w/Banana)	1	160	0	0	0	0	25	40	1
Sunrise Refresher	1	120	0	0	0	0	20	29	1

Soups (1 cup)

Food Item	Amount	Total Calories	Fat Calories	Total Fat (g)	Sat. Fat (g)	Chol. (mg)	Sodium (mg)	Carbo (g)	Protein (g)
Br. Wild Rice w/Chicken	1	190	100	11	4	20	990	17	6
Cheese/Ham/Bacon	1	240	140	15	6	20	1160	17	8
Chicken and Dumpling	1	130	40	4	2	30	1030	16	7
Chili Con Carne	1	240	90	10	5	15	860	23	15
Cream of Broccoli	1	130	50	6	0	10	860	15	5
Cream of Potato w/Bacon	1	200	100	11	4	15	840	21	4
Golden Broc. & Cheese	1	180	100	11	4	15	1120	16	5
Minestrone	1	90	35	4	1	20	1180	7	7

Food Item	Amount	Total Calories	Fat Calories	Total Fat (g)	Sat. Fat (g)	Chol. (mg)	Sodium (mg)	Carbo (g)	Protein (g)
New Eng. Clam Chowder	1	110	30	4	0	10	990	16	5
Roasted Chicken Noodle	1	60	15	2	0	10	940	7	6
Sp. Style Ch. with Rice	1	90	20	2	0	10	800	13	5
Tom. Gar. Veg. w/Rotini	1	100	5	0	0	0	900	20	3
Vegetable Beef	1	90	10	1	0	10	1050	15	5

Taco Bell®

Big Bell Value Menu

Food Item	Amount	Total Calories	Fat Calories	Total Fat (g)	Sat. Fat (g)	Chol. (mg)	Sodium (mg)	Carbo (g)	Protein (g)
Grande Soft Taco	1	450	190	21	8	45	1400	44	20
Double Decker Taco	1	340	120	14	5	25	800	39	15
1/2 lb. Bean Burrito Esp.	1	600	190	21	5	25	800	39	15
1/2 lb. Beef Combo Bur.	1	470	170	19	7	45	1610	52	22
1/2 lb. Beef/Potato Bur.	1	530	220	24	9	40	1670	65	15
Cheesy Fiesta Potatoes	1	280	160	18	6	20	800	27	4
Caramel Apple Empanada	1	290	130	15	4	5	290	37	3

Tacos

Food Item	Amount	Total Calories	Fat Calories	Total Fat (g)	Sat. Fat (g)	Chol. (mg)	Sodium (mg)	Carbo (g)	Protein (g)
Crunchy Taco	1	170	90	10	4	25	350	13	8
Taco Supreme	1	220	120	14	7	40	360	14	9
Soft Taco Beef	1	210	90	10	4.5	25	620	21	10
Ranchero Chicken Soft	1	270	130	15	4	35	790	21	13
Soft Taco Supreme Beef	1	260	130	14	7	40	630	22	11
Soft Taco Supreme Ch.	1	230	90	10	5	45	570	21	15
Grilled Steak Soft Taco	1	280	150	17	4.5	30	650	21	12
Double Decker Taco Sup.	1	380	160	18	8	40	820	40	15

Gorditas

Food Item	Amount	Total Calories	Fat Calories	Total Fat (g)	Sat. Fat (g)	Chol. (mg)	Sodium (mg)	Carbo (g)	Protein (g)
Supreme Beef	1	310	140	16	7	35	590	30	14
Supreme Chicken	1	290	110	12	5	45	530	28	17
Supreme Steak	1	290	120	13	6	35	520	28	16
Baja Beef	1	350	170	19	5	30	750	31	14
Baja Chicken	1	320	170	19	5	30	750	31	14
Baja Steak	1	320	150	16	4	30	680	29	15
Nacho Cheese Beef	1	300	120	13	4	20	740	32	13
Nacho Cheese Chicken	1	270	90	10	2.5	25	670	30	16
Nacho Cheese Steak	1	270	100	11	3	20	660	30	14

Chalupas

Food Item	Amount	Total Calories	Fat Calories	Total Fat (g)	Sat. Fat (g)	Chol. (mg)	Sodium (mg)	Carbo (g)	Protein (g)
Supreme Beef	1	390	220	24	10	40	600	31	14
Supreme Chicken	1	370	180	20	8	45	530	30	17
Supreme Steak	1	370	190	22	8	35	520	29	15
Baja Beef	1	430	250	27	8	30	750	32	14

Food Item	Amount	Total Calories	Fat Calories	Total Fat (g)	Sat. Fat (g)	Chol. (mg)	Sodium (mg)	Carbo (g)	Protein (g)
Baja Chicken	1	400	210	24	6	40	690	30	17
Baja Steak	1	400	220	25	7	30	680	30	15
Nacho Cheese Beef	1	380	200	22	7	20	740	33	12
Nacho Cheese Chicken	1	350	160	18	5	25	670	31	16
Nacho Cheese Steak	1	350	170	19	5	20	670	31	14

Burritos

Food Item	Amount	Total Calories	Fat Calories	Total Fat (g)	Sat. Fat (g)	Chol. (mg)	Sodium (mg)	Carbo (g)	Protein (g)
Bean	1	370	90	10	3.5	10	1200	55	14
7-Layer	1	530	190	21	8	25	1350	66	18
Chili Cheese	1	390	160	18	9	40	1080	40	16
Supreme Beef	1	440	160	18	8	40	1330	51	18
Supreme Chicken	1	410	130	14	6	45	1270	50	21
Supreme Steak	1	420	140	16	7	35	1260	50	19
Fiesta Beef	1	390	140	15	5	25	1150	50	14
Fiesta Chicken	1	370	100	12	3.5	30	1090	48	18
Fiesta Steak	1	370	110	13	4	25	1080	48	16
Grilled Stuft Beef	1	730	300	33	11	55	2080	79	28
Grilled Stuft Chicken	1	680	230	26	7	70	1950	76	35
Grilled Stuft Steak	1	680	250	28	8	55	1940	76	31

Specialties

Food Item	Amount	Total Calories	Fat Calories	Total Fat (g)	Sat. Fat (g)	Chol. (mg)	Sodium (mg)	Carbo (g)	Protein (g)
Tostada	1	250	90	10	4	15	710	29	11
Mexican Pizza	1	550	280	31	11	45	1030	46	21
Enchirito Beef	1	380	160	18	9	45	1430	35	19
Enchirito Chicken	1	350	130	14	7	55	1360	33	23
Enchirito Steak	1	360	140	16	8	45	1350	33	21
MexiMelt	1	290	140	16	8	45	880	23	15
Fiesta Taco Salad	1	870	430	48	16	65	1770	80	32
Fiesta Taco S. w/Shell	1	500	230	26	11	65	1520	42	25
Express Taco S. w/Chips	1	620	280	31	13	65	1390	60	27
Cheese Quesadilla	1	490	260	28	13	55	1150	39	19
Chicken Quesadilla	1	540	270	30	13	80	1380	40	28
Steak Quesadilla	1	540	280	31	14	70	1370	40	26
Zesty Ch. Border Bowl	1	730	380	42	9	45	1640	65	23
Zesty Ch. Bor. B. w/o Dress.	1	500	170	19	4.5	30	1400	60	22
Southwest Steak Bow	1	700	290	32	8	55	2050	73	30

Nachos and Sides

Food Item	Amount	Total Calories	Fat Calories	Total Fat (g)	Sat. Fat (g)	Chol. (mg)	Sodium (mg)	Carbo (g)	Protein (g)
Nachos	1	320	170	19	4.5	5	530	33	5
Nachos Supreme	1	460	230	26	9	35	800	42	13
Nachos BellGrande	1	780	380	43	13	35	1300	80	20
Pintos 'n Cheese	1	180	60	7	3.5	15	700	20	10
Mexican Rice	1	210	90	10	4	15	740	23	6
Cinnamon Twists	1	160	50	5	1	0	150	28	1

Food Item	Amount	Total Calories	Fat Calories	Total Fat (g)	Sat. Fat (g)	Chol. (mg)	Sodium (mg)	Carbo (g)	Protein (g)

Wendy's®

Sandwiches

Food Item	Amount	Total Calories	Fat Calories	Total Fat (g)	Sat. Fat (g)	Chol. (mg)	Sodium (mg)	Carbo (g)	Protein (g)
Classic Single w/Every.	1	410	170	19	7	70	920	37	25
Big Bacon Classic	1	580	270	30	12	100	1460	46	34
Jr. Hamburger	1	270	80	9	3	30	620	34	14
Jr. Cheeseburger	1	310	110	12	6	45	800	34	17
Jr. Bacon Cheeseburger	1	380	170	19	7	55	870	34	20
Jr. Cheeseburger Deluxe	1	350	140	16	6	50	860	36	18
Ultimate Chicken Grill	1	360	60	7	1.5	75	1100	44	31
Homestyle Ch. Fillet	1	540	190	22	4	55	1320	57	29
Spicy Chicken Fillet	1	510	170	19	3.5	55	1480	57	29

Side Selections

Food Item	Amount	Total Calories	Fat Calories	Total Fat (g)	Sat. Fat (g)	Chol. (mg)	Sodium (mg)	Carbo (g)	Protein (g)
Caesar Side Salad	1	70	40	4.5	2	10	190	2	6
Side Salad	1	35	0	0	0	0	20	7	2
Plain Baked Potato	1	270	0	0	0	0	25	61	7
Bacon & Cheese B. Potato	1	560	220	25	74	35	910	67	16
Broc. & Cheese B. Potato	1	440	130	15	3	10	540	70	10
Sour Cr. & Chive B. Pot.	1	340	60	6	4	15	40	62	8
Chili (small)	1	200	45	5	2	35	870	21	17
Chili (large)	1	300	70	7	3	50	1310	31	25
Shredded Cheddar Cheese	2 T.	70	50	6	3.5	15	110	1	4
Saltine Crackers	1 pkt.	25	5	0.5	0	0	80	4	1
French Fries (kids)	1	250	100	11	2	0	220	36	3
French Fries (medium)	1	390	150	17	3	0	340	56	4
French Fries (biggie)	1	440	170	19	3.5	0	380	63	5
French Fries (great biggie)	1	530	200	23	4.5	0	450	75	6

Homestyle Chicken Strips & Crispy Chicken Nuggets

Food Item	Amount	Total Calories	Fat Calories	Total Fat (g)	Sat. Fat (g)	Chol. (mg)	Sodium (mg)	Carbo (g)	Protein (g)
Homestyle Ch. Strips	3	410	160	18	3.5	60	1470	33	28
Deli Honey Must. Sauce	1	170	140	16	2.5	15	190	6	0
Spicy SW Chipotle Sauce	1	140	120	13	2	20	170	5	0
Heartland Ranch Sauce	1	200	190	21	3.5	20	280	1	0
Crispy Chicken Nuggets	4	180	100	11	2.5	25	390	10	8
Crispy Chicken Nuggets	5	220	130	14	3	35	490	13	10
Barbecue Sauce	1	40	0	0	0	0	160	10	1
Honey Mustard Sauce	1	130	100	12	2	10	220	6	0
Sweet and Sour Sauce	1	45	0	0	0	0	120	12	0

Garden Sensations Salads

Food Item	Amount	Total Calories	Fat Calories	Total Fat (g)	Sat. Fat (g)	Chol. (mg)	Sodium (mg)	Carbo (g)	Protein (g)
Mandarin Chicken	1	190	25	3	1	50	740	17	22
Crispy Noodles	1	60	20	2	0	0	170	10	1
Roasted Almonds	1	130	100	11	1	0	70	4	5

Food Item	Amount	Total Calories	Fat Calories	Total Fat (g)	Sat. Fat (g)	Chol. (mg)	Sodium (mg)	Carbo (g)	Protein (g)
Oriental Ses. Dr.	1	250	170	19	2.5	0	560	19	1
Spring Mix	1	180	100	11	6	30	230	12	11
Honey R. Pecans	1	130	120	13	12	0	65	5	2
House Vin. Dr.	1	190	160	18	2.5	0	730	8	0
Chicken BLT	1	360	170	19	9	95	1140	10	34
Home. Gar. Cr.	1	70	25	2.5	0	0	120	9	1
Honey Mus. Dr.	1	280	230	26	4	25	350	11	1
Taco Supreme	1	360	140	16	8	65	1090	29	27
Salsa	1	30	0	0	0	0	440	6	1
Sour Cream	1	60	45	5	305	20	20	2	1
Taco Chips	1	220	100	11	2	0	200	27	3
Homestyle Ch. Strips	1	450	200	22	9	70	1190	34	29
Creamy R. Dr.	1	230	200	23	4	15	580	5	1

Additional Salad Dressings

Food Item	Amount	Total Calories	Fat Calories	Total Fat (g)	Sat. Fat (g)	Chol. (mg)	Sodium (mg)	Carbo (g)	Protein (g)
Blue Cheese	1	360	350	38	7	30	350	1	2
French	1	250	190	21	3	0	670	13	0
French, Fat Free	1	70	0	0	0	0	300	18	0
Italian Caesar	1	230	220	24	4	25	350	1	1
Italian, Reduced Fat	1	80	60	7	1	0	690	6	0
Hidden Valley Ranch	1	200	180	20	3	25	410	3	1
H. Val. Ran. Dr., Red, Fat	1	120	100	11	2	20	470	4	1
Thousand Island	1	260	230	25	4	20	380	7	1

Frosty

Food Item	Amount	Total Calories	Fat Calories	Total Fat (g)	Sat. Fat (g)	Chol. (mg)	Sodium (mg)	Carbo (g)	Protein (g)
Junior	1	170	40	4	2.5	20	100	26	4
Small	1	330	80	8	5	35	200	56	8
Medium	1	440	100	11	7	50	260	73	11

CINNAMON CREAM CHEESE TRIANGLES

20 calories

Makes 64 appetizer triangles—20 calories per triangle

- 8 oz. cream cheese, softened
- ¼ cup soft silken tofu
- 1 tsp. cinnamon
- 1 T. Splenda or granular alternative sweetener
- ⅔ cup finely chopped pecans
- 32 slices thin sliced whole wheat bread

In a small bowl, combine the first 5 ingredients. Cut crusts from bread, if desired. Spread half the bread slices with the cream cheese mixture; top each with second bread slice. Cut each diagonally twice, making an "X." This will make 4 appetizer triangles from each sandwich.

STUFFED APRICOTS

50 calories

Makes about 5 dozen stuffed apricots—50 calories per 4 apricots

- 5 dozen dried apricots (about 1¼ cups)

Filling

- 8 oz. cream cheese
- ½ cup silken tofu
- 1 tsp. cinnamon
- ½ tsp. ground ginger
- ½ tsp. ground nutmeg
- 1 T. Whey Low (fructose, agave nectar, or Splenda may be used)
- ¼ cup finely chopped walnuts

Using a narrow knife, such as a paring knife, make a slit on the end of each apricot, twisting the knife to open the inside. Set aside. Mix cream cheese, tofu, spices, and sweetener together. Place the mixture in a pastry bag, using a wider tip. Pipe the cream cheese mixture into each apricot. Dip the cream cheese end of each apricot into the finely chopped nuts. Arrange on tray; refrigerate until ready to serve.

CHEESE STRAWS

181 calories

Makes 6 dozen—181 calories per 4 straws

- 1 cup butter, softened
- 2 cups shredded, extra sharp cheese, room temperature
- 1¾ cups whole wheat or spelt flour (fluff with spoon before measuring)
- ½ tsp. salt
- ½ tsp. ground cayenne pepper
- 1 tsp. lemon juice

Preheat the oven to 300°F. Using a mixer, beat the butter at medium speed until creamy. Gradually add the cheese, beating well. Add flour, salt, and pepper. Beat at low speed until blended. Add lemon juice and beat for 15 minutes at medium speed. Pipe the mixture from a pastry bag or drop dough by teaspoonfuls onto ungreased baking sheets. Bake for about 12 minutes, until set. Cool on wire racks.

DILLED DEVILED EGGS

99 calories

Serves 8 to 12—99 calories for 2 halves

- 1 dozen large eggs
- ¼ cup sugar-free mayonnaise
- 2 T. white wine vinegar
- 1 tsp. dry mustard
- ¼ tsp. salt
- dash black pepper
- ¼ tsp. dried dill
- paprika

Cover the eggs with cold water in a medium saucepan. Bring to a boil; reduce heat to medium, so that the water remains at a low boil. Boil for 15 minutes. Immediately drain water and place eggs in cold water. Crack the shells and peel. If you do not do this immediately, the eggs will be difficult to peel. Slice the eggs in half lengthwise; remove the yolks to a medium bowl. Arrange the whites on a platter. To the yolks, add mayonnaise, mustard, salt, pepper, dill weed, and vinegar. Mix with a fork until smooth and creamy. With a teaspoon, fill the whites with the yolk mixture. Lightly sprinkle the paprika. Refrigerate until ready to serve.

FRUIT & NUT TABOULI

100 calories

Serves 8—100 calories per serving

- 1¼ cups boiling water
- ½ cup bulgur (specialty grains and health food section of your grocery)
- 2 T. lemon juice
- ½ cup dried cranberries
- 1 apple, peeled, cored, and finely chopped (about 1 cup)
- 2 T. olive oil
- ¼ cup minced onion
- ¼ cup finely chopped walnuts
- ½ cucumber, peeled, seeded, and finely chopped
- ¼ cup finely chopped celery with tops
- 1 tsp. grated fresh ginger
- ¼ tsp. salt

Measure the bulgur into a bowl; pour the boiling water over and cover with a plate for 20 minutes. While waiting, put the lemon juice into a large bowl and add the cranberries. Peel, core, and chop the apple. Add the lemon juice and toss together. Add all remaining ingredients, except the bulgur. After 20 minutes of steeping, drain the bulgur in a finely meshed strainer, gently pressing out the excess moisture. Add to the bowl of ingredients and serve. This dish is nice served freshly warm, at room temperature, or cold the next day.

SUMMER PEACH SALSA

Serves 6 to 8

- 1 jicama, peeled and sliced
- juice of 1 lime
- 1 to 2 ripe peaches, diced (about 1 cup)
- ½ cup fresh blueberries
- ½ sweet onion, minced
- ¼ tsp. freshly grated ginger

Pour the lime juice into a medium bowl. Peel and dice the peaches and add to the bowl, tossing to coat the peaches. Add the remaining ingredients and combine all. Place in pretty bowl and serve with jicama slices for dipping.

GRILLED PORTOBELLO MUSHROOMS

Serves 3 to 6

- 12 oz. thickly sliced portobello mushrooms
- 2 T. olive oil
- 1 clove garlic, crushed
- ¼ tsp. salt
- pepper to taste

Heat the grill. Combine all ingredients except the mushrooms. Brush the mushrooms with the oil mixture. Place on a hot grill, turning after 5 minutes or until the heated side is crisp.

Alternative cooking method.
Heat a nonstick skillet on medium-high. Add mushrooms that have been brushed with oil and braise until crispy on both sides.

BLACK BEAN CAKES

259
calories

Makes 6 (4") cakes—259 calories per cake

- 2 (15 oz.) cans black beans, rinsed and drained
- 2 eggs, beaten
- 1 small onion, minced
- 1 clove garlic, crushed
- ½ tsp. salt
- ¼ tsp. ground cumin
- dash Tabasco
- 2 T. whole wheat flour
- ¼ cup + 1 T. canola oil, divided

In a small pan, sauté the onion until translucent. Add garlic and continue to sauté for 1 minute. Set aside. In medium bowl, lightly mash beans until broken, but not pasty. Add all other ingredients, including the onions and mix gently. In a large skillet, preheat ¼" of oil in pan on medium-high (until a drop of water sizzles when added). Drop the bean mixture by large spoonfuls into hot oil; flatten gently with second spoon or spatula. Cook about 5 minutes per side, turning once. Cakes should be lightly browned. Drain on paper towels. Serve with sour cream and salsa.

GINGERED WATERMELON & YELLOW TOMATO SALAD

130 calories

Serves 6—130 calories per serving

- 4 lb. piece of watermelon, preferably seedless
- 2 lb. vine-ripened tomatoes, preferably yellow
- 1 tsp. coarse salt, preferably sea salt
- ½ small red onion
- 2 T. fresh lime juice
- 1 tsp. finely grated peeled fresh gingerroot
- ½ tsp. sugar

Remove rind and any seeds from watermelon. Cut the fruit into 1½" pieces and put into a large bowl. Cut the tomatoes into 1½" pieces. Add tomatoes and salt to watermelon, tossing to combine. Let mixture stand at cool room temperature for 3 hours.

In a colander set over a small saucepan, drain the mixture and transfer to a bowl. Simmer liquid until reduced to about 2 T. and cool completely. Halve the onion and thinly slice enough to measure ¼ cup. Add onion to watermelon mixture. For best results do not chill salad as it will lose flavor. In a small bowl stir together reduced watermelon-tomato juice, lime juice, gingerroot, and sugar. Just before serving, toss salad with juice mixture.

CANTALOUPE WITH BLACK PEPPER, VINEGAR, & CHIVES SALAD

30 calories

Serves 4 to 6—30 calories per serving

- ½ ripe cantaloupe, seeds removed
- 1 bunch of frisee (a type of curly endive)
- salt and freshly ground black pepper
- 2 tsp. white wine vinegar, preferably champagne vinegar
- 2 tsp. snipped fresh chives

With a melon baller, scoop out 1" balls from the melon and turn into a medium bowl. Place several leaves of washed and trimmed on individual salad plates. Sprinkle the melon with salt and pepper to taste. Toss gently with the vinegar. Spoon onto greens, scatter the chives over the melon and serve.

WATERCRESS, CHICORY, AND RADISH SALAD WITH BEET VINAIGRETTE

40 calories

Serves 4—40 calories per serving

- 1 chicory heart, torn into pieces
- 2 medium red radishes, thinly sliced
- 4 cups tightly packed watercress, tough stems removed
- 1/4 cup beet vinaigrette (recipe follows)
- salt and freshly ground black pepper

Reserve a handful of the chicory and about a quarter of the radishes. In a medium bowl, combine the watercress, the remaining chicory, and the remaining radishes. Add the vinaigrette and toss to coat. Season with the salt and pepper. Place equal portions on each of 4 salad plates. Scatter the reserved chicory and radishes over the top.

Beet Vinaigrette

- 3 oz. beets, cooked, peeled, and chopped
- 3/4 cup chicken stock (or 3/4 cup fresh squeezed orange juice)
- 1 tsp. olive oil
- 1 tsp. red wine vinegar
- salt and freshly ground black pepper

In a blender or a food processor fitted with a metal blade, combine the beets, stock, oil, and vinegar. Process until very smooth. Season with salt and pepper. Can be refrigerated for up to 2 days.

INDONESIAN RICE SALAD WITH LIME DRESSING

210 calories

Serves 8—210 calories per serving

- 2 cups long-grain brown rice
- 4½ cups water
- lime dressing (recipe follows)
- 1/3 lb. snow peas, ends and strings removed
- 1 medium red bell pepper, seeded and chopped
- 5 green onions, thinly sliced
- 1 can (about 8 oz.) water chestnuts, drained and chopped
- 1/4 cup chopped cilantro
- 1/4 cup raisins (optional)

In a 3-quart pan, combine rice and water. Bring to boil over high heat, cover, and simmer until rice is tender to the bite (about 45 minutes). Let cool, uncovered, in pan. Meanwhile, prepare the lime dressing.

Lime dressing

In a small bowl, mix ⅔ cup rice or cider vinegar, 2 T. each reduced-sodium soy sauce and lime juice, and 2 tsp. minced garlic.

Thinly slice the snow peas. Place in a large bowl; add the red pepper, onions, water chestnuts, cilantro, raisins (if desired), rice, and lime dressing. Mix to blend. Spoon salad into a shallow serving bowl.

SPICY CHICKEN & ORANGE SALAD

290 calories

Serves 4—290 calories per serving

- cilantro dressing (recipe follows)
- 5 large oranges
- about 30 large spinach leaves, rinsed
- 1 lb. skinless chicken breasts, cut into ½" wide strips
- 1 T. minced garlic
- 1 tsp. each chili powder and dried oregano
- 1 tsp. reduced-sodium soy sauce
- cilantro sprigs
- ¼ tsp. curry powder

Prepare cilantro dressing; set aside. Peel oranges and cut crosswise into thin slices. Arrange a fourth of the orange slices and spinach leaves on 4 salad or dinner plates. Lightly film a wide frying pan with vegetable oil or cooking spray. Over high heat add chicken strips, garlic, chili, and oregano. Cook, stirring, until chicken is no longer pink in the center (about 5 minutes). Add cilantro dressing and soy sauce; stir. Spoon hot chicken mixture equally over oranges. Garnish with cilantro sprigs.

Cilantro dressing

In a bowl, mix ½ cup lime juice, 2 T. sugar, and ¼ cup chopped cilantro.

SUMMER MINESTRONE

105 calories

Serves 6 to 8—105 calories per serving

- 2 tightly packed tsp. fresh basil leaves
- ¼ tightly packed fresh marjoram leaves
- leaves of 1 branch fresh thyme
- 3 scallions, thinly sliced
- 1 medium onion, cut into ⅛" dice
- 2 small carrots, cut into ⅛" dice
- 2 medium zucchini, cut into ⅛" dice
- 1 cup thinly sliced sugar snap peas (about ¼ lb.)
- 1 basket (¾ to 1 lb.) cherry tomatoes, cut into quarters
- salt and freshly ground pepper
- 5 cups canned low-sodium chicken broth

Mince together the herbs. Blend with the sliced scallions and set aside. Lightly film a 4-quart saucepan with olive oil or cooking spray and heat over medium high heat. Drop in the onion, carrots, zucchini, peas, and half the tomatoes. Sprinkle with salt and pepper and sauté for 3 minutes or until the vegetables are wilted. Add the broth and boil 5 minutes or until the vegetables are tender-crisp (do not cover). Stir in a quarter of the herb mixture and remove the soup from the heat. Serve hot, warm, or at room temperature, topping each serving with some of the remaining tomatoes and the herb blend.

GINGERED CARROT SOUP

35 calories

Serves 6—35 calories per serving

- ½ cup onion, finely chopped
- 2 cloves garlic, minced
- 5 cups carrots, thinly sliced
- 1 T. fresh ginger, minced
- 4 cups low-sodium chicken stock
- ¼ cup lime juice
- pinch of curry
- chives, chopped
- fat-free yogurt (optional)

Lightly film a heavy pot with olive oil or cooking spray. Over medium-low heat, add onion and sauté until tender but not browned, about 10 minutes. Add garlic and cook 3 minutes more. Stir in carrots and ginger. Add chicken stock and simmer until carrots are tender, about 20 minutes. Add lime juice and curry and puree soup in blender until smooth. Chill or serve warm, topped with a dollop of yogurt, if desired, and a sprinkle of chives.

MEXICAN GAZPACHO

60 calories

Serves 6—60 calories per serving

- 1½ lb. ripe tomatoes, peeled, seeded, and chopped (about 2 cups)
- ¼ cup chopped red onion
- ¼ cup chopped celery
- 3 T. chopped scallion
- ¼ cup chopped sweet green pepper
- ½ cup cucumber cut into ¼" cubes (or very coarsely chopped in a food processor)
- 2 T. chopped green hot or mild chilies
- 1 T. chopped garlic
- ¼ cup chopped cilantro
- 2 T. chopped Italian parsley
- 1 cup tomato juice
- 2 T. red wine vinegar
- 2 T. fresh lime juice
- ½ tsp. salt
- freshly ground black pepper, to taste

Combine all the ingredients in a mixing bowl, cover the bowl with plastic wrap, and refrigerate until cold. Serve the soup in large chilled bowls.

CUCUMBER & MINT SOUP

70 calories

Serves 4 to 6—70 calories per serving

- 2 cucumbers (2 lb. total), peeled, seeded, and coarsely chopped
- ¼ cup (loosely packed) mint leaves
- 3 cloves garlic, peeled
- 1¼ cups cold water
- 1½ cups nonfat yogurt
- 2 T. cider vinegar
- 1½ tsp. salt
- 10 drops Tabasco hot pepper sauce

Place the cucumber chunks in the bowl of a food processor with the mint, garlic, and ½ cup of cold water. Process until pureed; the mixture will be granular. (For a smoother texture, puree in a conventional blender or with a handheld immersion blender.) Transfer the puree to a bowl and mix in the yogurt, vinegar, salt, Tabasco, and remaining ¾ cup of water. Chill. Stir before serving.

CHUNKY VEGETABLE SOUP

195 calories

Serves 12—195 calories per serving

- 1 cup chopped onions
- 1 T. chopped garlic
- 2 cups diced ripe tomatoes
- 2 cups zucchini cut in ½" cubes
- 1 cup carrots cut into ¼" cubes
- 1 cup white turnips cut into ¼" cubes
- 1 cup chopped celery
- 1 lb. dried navy beans
- freshly ground black pepper
- 10 cups low-sodium chicken stock
- ¼ cup chopped fresh basil leaves
- salt, if necessary

Lightly film the bottom of a soup kettle with olive oil or coat with a cooking spray. Add the onion and garlic. Cook them briefly and add the tomatoes, zucchini, carrots, turnips, and celery. Stir for about 10 minutes. Add the beans, pepper, and stock. Bring to a boil and simmer for about 1 hour 45 minutes. Add the basil and salt, if desired.

GRILLED CHICKEN PIECES IN SICILIAN MINT SAUCE

290 calories

Serves 4—290 calories per serving

Chicken
- 4 skinless, boneless chicken breasts, cut crosswise into 1/2" strips
- shredded zest of 1 medium lemon
- 1/2 tsp. dried oregano
- 1/8 tsp. freshly ground black pepper
- salt

Mint Sauce
- 1/4 medium red onion, minced
- 1 clove garlic, minced
- generous pinch of sugar
- 3 T. white or red wine vinegar
- salt and freshly ground black pepper
- 1 T. extra virgin olive oil
- 1/4 tightly packed cup fresh mint leaves, finely chopped

Toss the chicken with the lemon zest, oregano, and pepper. Marinate in the refrigerator 1 to 6 hours. About 30 minutes before cooking, stir together the minced onion, garlic, sugar, vinegar, and salt and pepper to taste in a small bowl. Let stand 20 minutes, then whisk in oil. About 15 minutes before serving, heat a 12" nonstick sauté pan over medium-high heat. Sauté the chicken, sprinkling it with salt. Turn the pieces as they pick up color and immediately reduce the heat to medium-low. Continue cooking about 5 minutes, stirring occasionally, or until chicken is barely firm when pressed; be sure there is no sign of raw meat. Transfer the chicken to a serving platter. Stir 3 T. of fresh mint into the sauce. Taste for seasoning, then spoon over the chicken. Sprinkle the remaining mint over the dish just before serving.

SPICY SUMMER CHICKEN STIR-FRY

280 calories

Serves 6 to 8—280 calories per serving

- 3 whole skinless, boneless chicken breasts (about 2½ lb. total), cut into 1" to 2" strips about ½" wide
- ¾ tsp. salt
- 1 small onion, sliced, separated into rings
- 2 or 3 cloves garlic, minced
- 2 zucchini, each about 6" long and 1½" in diameter, thinly sliced
- 2 yellow crookneck squash, each about 6" long and 1½" in diameter, thinly sliced
- 6 fresh new Mexico hot green chilies, parched, peeled, seeded, chopped
- ¼ cup chopped fresh cilantro

Sprinkle chicken with salt and stir together. Lightly coat a wok or heavy skillet with olive oil or cooking spray and heat to medium-high. Add chicken strips and stir-fry until meat begins to lose its pink color. Then push the chicken to one side, away from the hot center of the pan. Add onion and stir-fry until it barely begins to get limp; then add the garlic, zucchini, and crookneck squash. Stir-fry 2 to 3 minutes or until color of squash heightens. Add chilies and cilantro; stir chicken back into the center of the pan. Stir-fry until chicken is done and squash is still slightly crisp.

GRILLED CHIPOTLE-MARINATED PORK

240 calories

Serves 4—240 calories per serving

- 2 (10 oz.) pork tenderloins, trimmed of all fat
- 3 canned chipotle chilies in adobo sauce, seeded
- 2 T. lime juice
- 3 T. honey
- 2 large cloves garlic
- 1 T. soy sauce
- 2 tsp. ground cumin
- ¼ cup chopped fresh cilantro plus sprigs for garnish

Cut each tenderloin in half crosswise. Set aside. In a blender, combine the chipotle chilies, lime juice, honey, garlic, soy sauce, and cumin and blend until smooth. Stir in cilantro. Transfer half of the mixture to a shallow, non-aluminum bowl. Reserve the other half. Add the pork to the bowl and turn to coat. Cover and refrigerate for 4 to 6 hours.

Prepare a fire in a grill or preheat a griddle over medium-high heat. Coat the grill rack about 6" to 8" from the fire or on the griddle. Cook until seared on the first side, about 4 minutes. Turn over the pork and spoon the reserved chili mixture evenly on the top of the pieces. Tent them with aluminum foil. Continue to cook until the pork is just firm to the touch and pale pink when cut into the thickest point, about 4 minutes longer. Transfer to a cutting board and let cool for about 8 minutes. Slice and arrange on warmed individual plates. Garnish with cilantro sprigs and serve hot.

GRILLED SHRIMP WITH LIME-CILANTRO MARINADE

95
calories

Serves 6 to 8—95 calories per serving

- 1 large bunch of fresh cilantro
- 8 medium-large chopped scallions
- 2 green chilies (the heat is up to you)
- 2 tsp. minced garlic
- 1 T. lime juice
- 2 tsp. ground cumin
- pinch of turmeric
- 3 lb. large shrimp

For garnish
- coarse salt
- freshly ground black pepper
- ancho chili powder
- lime quarters
- fresh cilantro

In a blender or food processor place the cilantro leaves and stems, scallions, chilies, garlic, lime juice, cumin, and turmeric. Puree, adding a little water if necessary to achieve the desired consistency. Peel the shrimp, leaving the tail intact. De-vein them, place them in a glass bowl, and toss with the cilantro puree. Marinate 8 to 12 hours.

Prepare a moderately hot charcoal fire. When ready to cook, scoop up the shrimp so that more of the marinade remains on one side of each one. Place the shrimp marinade-side up on the grill. Cook until almost done, about 2 minutes. Turn shrimp over and cook quickly on marinade side, about 1 minute. Remove shrimp from the grill and divide among serving plates. Pass garnishes at the table.

WHOLE TILAPIA WITH ONION AND LEMON

Serves 2—205 calories per serving

- 1¼ lb. red onions, thinly sliced
- 3 T. lemon juice
- 1 T. minced fresh ginger
- 1 whole tilapia, dressed
- 2 large lemons
- 3 T. minced cilantro
- salt and pepper

In a glass or ceramic bowl, mix onions, lemon juice, and ginger. Set 1 or 2 onions slices aside, then spread remaining onion mixture in a 9" x 13" glass or ceramic baking dish. Rinse fish, pat dry, and place on top of the onion mixture. Cut a ½" slice from both sides of each lemon. Stuff the fish cavity with these lemon ends, reserved onion slices, and 1½ T. of the cilantro. Thinly slice the remainder of each lemon and tuck lemon around fish. Sprinkle remaining 1½ T. cilantro over the onion mixture and lemon slices. Bake in 400°F oven until fish is just opaque but still moist in the thickest part; cut to test (about 20 minutes). Gently pull skin from fish and serve with the onion-lemon mixture. Season with salt and pepper.

GRILLED BUTTERFLIED LEG OF LAMB

Serves 10—161 calories per 3-oz. serving

- 2 T. minced fresh thyme
- 2 T. minced fresh rosemary
- 2 cloves garlic, minced
- 2 T. Dijon mustard
- 2 T. red wine vinegar
- freshly ground black pepper
- 1 leg of lamb (4 lb. boned), butterflied and trimmed of all fat
- coarse salt

In a small bowl, combine the thyme, rosemary, garlic, mustard, and vinegar. Generously season with the pepper. Rub the herb marinade over the lamb. Place the lamb in a large shallow container just large enough to hold it. Pour any remaining marinade over the top. Cover and refrigerate for at least 8 hours. Adjust the rack of the grill so that it is at least 10" above the heat source. Preheat the grill to medium.

Remove the lamb from the refrigerator. Uncover and generously season with salt. Place the lamb on the grill, cover and grill for 15 minutes. Turn the lamb, cover and grill for 15 minutes. Continue grilling to the desired doneness (about 10 additional minutes for rare; 15 to 20 minutes for medium). Throughout the grilling period, check the lamb to make sure that it is cooking slowly and not charring. If it does begin to burn, move the lamb away from the greatest heat.

Place the lamb on a carving board or serving platter. Let stand for 10 minutes. Cut across the grain into thin slices. Serve warm or at room temperature.

BLACK BEAN CHILI WITH EGGPLANT

205
calories

Serves 4—205 calories per serving

- 1½ lb. eggplant, unpeeled, stemmed, and cut into 1" cubes
- salt for sprinkling the eggplant plus additional to taste
- 15 dried New Mexican red chilies (about 3 oz.)
- 3 cups water
- 2 small red onions, finely chopped
- 4 garlic cloves, minced
- 28-oz. can plum tomatoes, drained and chopped
- ½ T. ground coriander
- ½ tsp. ground cumin
- 1 bay leaf
- 2 cups cooked black beans

Garnish

- red onions, finely diced
- cilantro, coarsely chopped

Place the eggplant cubes into a strainer and sprinkle generously with salt. Let stand for 1 hour and pat dry with a paper towel. Simmer the chilies and the 3 cups of water in a large saucepan for 20 minutes. Puree the chilies and the liquid, in batches, in a blender until very smooth. Force the puree through the fine sieve and discard any solid pieces. Lightly film a large, heavy Dutch oven with olive oil or cooking spray, add eggplant, and cook, stirring over moderately high heat, until almost tender (about 4 minutes). Remove eggplant and set aside. Re-film the Dutch oven with oil if necessary and add onions and garlic. Cook, stirring, for 4 minutes. Add tomatoes, ground coriander, cumin, bay leaf, eggplant, and chili puree, and simmer for 5 minutes. Add beans and simmer over moderate heat for 15 minutes. Season to taste with salt. Remove the bay leaf. Place in bowls and top with onions and cilantro.

FISH FILLETS WITH TOMATO-CILANTRO SALSA

Serves 6

Salsa

- 8 plum tomatoes, seeded and diced (about 2⅔ cup)
- 1 red onion, diced (about 1 cup)
- 1 bunch fresh cilantro, chopped (about ½ cup)
- ¼ cup fresh lime juice
- 1 T. olive oil
- 2 tsp. minced canned chipotle chilies
- ½ tsp. ground cumin

Fish

- 3 T. olive oil
- 6 (6 oz.) tilapia or orange roughy fillets (each about ¾" thick)
- 1 lb. tender, slim green beans, trimmed
- fresh lemon juice
- additional olive oil

To prepare the salsa, toss all ingredients into a large bowl to combine. Cover and refrigerate. Can be made up to 4 hours ahead.

To prepare the fish, preheat the over to 450°F. Brush both sides of the fish with olive oil, sprinkle with salt and pepper, then bake 8 to 10 minutes, or until done.

Meanwhile, cook the beans in a large pot of boiling water until crisp-tender, about 3 minutes. Drain and transfer to ice water to cool; drain. Season to taste with lemon juice and olive oil. Divide beans equally among plates. Top with fish fillets and salsa.

GRILLED SALMON WITH LEMON-GINGER MARINADE

Serves 6

- 8 (6 oz.) fillets of salmon, rinsed in cold water and patted dry
- salt and fresh ground pepper, to taste
- vegetable oil, as needed
- 2 oz. freshly chopped parsley
- 2 lemons, cut into wedges

Lemon-Ginger Marinade

- 8 oz. freshly squeezed lemon juice, strained
- 3 cloves garlic, peeled and finely diced
- 2 oz. fresh ginger root, peeled and finely diced
- 1 oz. fresh thyme, washed, leaves removed and chopped
- 2 oz. scallions, washed, trimmed, and cut into ¼" rings

GRILLED SALMON WITH LEMON-GINGER MARINADE CONTINUED

Combine the ingredients for the marinade and mix well. Season the salmon fillets with salt and pepper and place in a pan. Pour the marinade over the fish and refrigerate for 30 minutes. Turn once in marinade. Preheat the grill or broiler. Remove the fish from the marinade and pat each dry. Brush the fillets with oil. Grill the fish until seared and then brush the fish with marinade and turn. Grill until the fish is firm and opaque. Strain the remaining juice from the marinade through a small strainer into a small pot and bring to a boil. Reduce to the desired strength. To serve, place a fillet on a preheated dinner plate, spoon the juice from the marinade over the fillet, and garnish with parsley and a lemon wedge.

CARAMELIZED VEAL CHOPS WITH BALSAMIC SYRUP

Serves 4

- $1/3$ cup balsamic vinegar
- 2 T. soy sauce
- $1/2$ cup orange juice
- 1 T. sugar
- 2 tsp. crushed white peppercorns
- 4 (6 oz.) veal rib chops, trimmed of fat

In a small saucepan over medium-high heat, combine the vinegar and soy sauce. Bring to a boil, and boil until the liquid is reduced to 3 T., about 5 minutes. Remove from the heat, stir in the orange juice, and set aside.

In a small bowl, stir together the sugar and peppercorns. Press the sugar mixture onto one side of each veal chop, dividing it equally. Heat a large nonstick frying pan over medium-high heat. Coat the pan with nonstick cooking spray. Add the chops, sugar sides down, and cook until caramelized on the first side, about 2 minutes. Turn and continue to cook until pale pink when cut into at the thickest point, about 3 minutes longer. Transfer the chops to a warmed platter. Return the pan to medium-high heat. Pour in the reduced vinegar mixture and deglaze the pan, stirring with a wooden spoon to remove any browned bits from the pan bottom. Bring to a boil, and boil until the liquid is reduced to 3 tablespoons, about 3 minutes. Place chops on individual plates and top with the reduction. Garnish with orange slices or orange zest. Serve hot.

GRILLED FISH MADEIRA STYLE

Serves 2

Sauce

- 2 ripe tomatoes
- 1 tsp. olive oil
- ¼ cup finely chopped onion
- 1 medium clove garlic, peeled and minced
- ¼ cup dry white wine
- 1 bay leaf
- ½ tsp. paprika
- ⅛ tsp. cayenne pepper
- ¼ tsp. salt
- freshly ground pepper to taste
- 2 T. chopped parsley

Fish

- ½ to ⅔ lb. salmon fillet
- ½ tsp. olive oil
- ¼ tsp. paprika
- ⅛ tsp. cayenne pepper
- ⅛ tsp. salt
- freshly ground black pepper to taste

To prepare the sauce: Core the tomatoes. Bring a small pan of water to the boil, add the tomatoes and time 30 seconds to 1 minute, until the skins start to crack. Drain, peel, and coarsely chop the tomatoes. Heat the olive oil in a nonstick skillet. Add the onion and garlic, sauté 5 minutes. Add the tomatoes, wine, bay leaf, paprika, cayenne, salt, and pepper. Bring to a boil, reduce the heat, and simmer 20 minutes. Stir in the parsley at the end of the cooking time.

To prepare the fish: Place the fish on an oiled grill. Brush with the olive oil; sprinkle with the paprika, cayenne, salt, and pepper. Cook over medium coals in a covered grill 14 minutes per inch of thickness. The fish can also be baked in a preheated 450°F oven 12 minutes per inch of thickness. Test the fish for doneness. Serve the fish with the sauce on the side.

Note: The fish can also be served simply without the sauce and with a wedge of lemon.

HALIBUT ANTIBOISE

Serves 4

- 4 pieces halibut, skin removed and cleaned of sinews, each about 6 oz. and ¾" thick (1½ lb.)
- ½ tsp. salt
- 1 tsp. virgin olive oil

Antiboise Sauce

- 2 T. extra virgin olive oil
- ½ cup chopped onion
- 1 tsp. chopped fresh thyme leaves
- 2 tomatoes (12 oz. total), peeled, seeded, and cut in ½" pieces (1½ cups)
- ¼ cup water
- ½ tsp. salt
- ¼ tsp. freshly ground black pepper
- 24 Kalamata olives, pitted and cut into ½" pieces (½ cup)
- 2 T. shredded basil

For the sauce: Heat the 2 T. olive oil in a skillet. Add the onion and thyme. Cook over medium heat for 1½ minutes, then add the tomatoes, water, ½ tsp. salt, and pepper. Cook for 1 minute longer, then set the sauce aside. (The sauce can be prepared to this point up to 2 hours ahead.) Reserve the olives and basil in separate bowls for last minute addition to the sauce.

About 15 minutes before serving time, preheat the broiler. At serving time, sprinkle both sides of the halibut steaks with the ½ tsp. salt and brush them with the tsp. of olive oil. Arrange the steaks on a cookie sheet (lined, if desired, with aluminum foil), and place it under the hot broiler so the steaks are about 4" from the heat. Cook the steaks about 3 minutes on each side or until cooked through. Arrange the steak on each of four warmed dinner plates. Add the reserved olives and basil to the sauce and bring the mixture to a boil. Pour the sauce over the steaks and serve immediately.

SEARED SCALLOPS WITH TROPICAL SALSA

- 1/2 cup diced pineapple
- 1/2 cup diced mango
- 1/2 cup diced cucumber
- 1/2 cup diced red bell pepper
- 3 T. chopped fresh cilantro
- 4 tsp. fresh lime juice
- 1 jalapeno chili, seeded and minced
- salt and pepper to taste
- 16 sea scallops, about 1 lb.

In a bowl, combine the pineapple, mango, cucumber, bell pepper, cilantro, lime juice, and chili. Toss well to form a salsa. Season to taste with salt and pepper. Set aside.

Heat a large nonstick frying pan over medium-high heat. Coat the pan with nonstick cooking spray. Season the scallops with salt and pepper. Add half of the scallops to the pan and sear, turning once, until golden brown on both sides and opaque throughout, about 2 minutes on each side. (Be careful not to overcook as scallops will become rubbery.) Transfer scallops to a warmed plate. Keep warm while cooking the remaining scallops in the same way. Divide the scallops among warmed individual plates. Spoon the salsa over the tops, dividing it evenly. Serve immediately.

TURKEY CHILI

Serves 8

- 1 to 1 1/2 lbs. lean ground turkey
- 1 onion, minced
- 1 T. olive oil
- 2 to 3 cloves of garlic, crushed
- 1 sweet red pepper, halved, seeded and diced
- 1 sweet yellow pepper, halved, seeded and diced
- 1 large tin of whole or crushed tomatoes
- 3 to 4 cans (14 1/2 oz.) chicken stock
- chili powder to taste
- 2 pinches dried oregano
- 1/3 cup minced Italian parsley
- 1/3 cup minced cilantro
- 1 can kidney beans, drained
- 1 can black beans, drained
- 2 cans spicy chili beans, undrained
- salt and pepper to taste

Add oil to a heavy soup pan and brown the turkey and the onion, breaking up the meat with a spatula or spoon as it cooks. Add the garlic and the red and yellow pepper and let simmer for several minutes. Add the chicken stock, tomatoes, chili powder, and oregano. Cover and gently simmer for 1 to 2 hours. Just before serving add the cans of beans. Salt and pepper to taste. Heat through and serve.

Side Dishes

RATATOUILLE-TOPPED BAKED POTATOES

280 calories

Serves 6—280 calories per serving

- 1 medium-size eggplant (about 1 lb.), peeled, cut into 1/2" x 2" sticks
- 8 oz. each zucchini and crookneck squash, cut into 1/2" thick slices
- 1 1/2 lbs. Roma tomatoes, quartered
- 1 each large red and yellow peppers, seeded and thinly sliced
- 1 large onion, chopped
- 3 garlic cloves, minced or pressed
- 1 dry bay leaf
- 1/2 tsp. each dried thyme and dried rosemary
- 1 T. freshly squeezed lemon juice
- 6 large baking potatoes
- freshly ground pepper

In a 3- to 4-quart baking dish, mix the eggplant, zucchini, peppers, onion, garlic, bay leaf, rhyme, rosemary, and lemon juice. Cover and bake in a 400°F oven for 1 hour. Uncover and continue to bake, stirring once or twice, until eggplant is very soft when pressed and only a thin layer of liquid remains in the bottom of the dish (about 30 minutes more). After eggplant mixture has baked for the first 30 minutes, pierce each unpeeled potato in several places with a fork; place potatoes on a baking sheet and bake until tender throughout (about 1 hour). To serve, make a deep cut lengthwise down the center of each potato; then make a second cut across the center. Grasp each potato between cuts; press firmly to split potato wide open. Spoon eggplant mixture equally into potatoes; season to taste with pepper.

GRILLED TOMATOES

20 calories

Serves 12—20 calories per serving

- 6 large ripe tomatoes
- olive oil
- fresh thyme, minced
- salt and freshly ground black pepper

Halve the tomatoes crosswise. Gently squeeze each half to remove the seeds. Lightly brush the tomatoes with the oil. Place, cut size down, on the hottest part of the grill. Grill for 1 minute. Turn the tomatoes and move to the edge of the grill or wherever the heat is least hot. Grill for 3 minutes or until charred. Remove from the grill and season with the thyme and salt and pepper. Serve warm or at room temperature.

ROASTED ROOT VEGETABLES

60 calories

Serves 8 to 10—60 calories per serving

- 1 (2½ lb.) butternut squash, peeled, seeded, cut into ½" pieces
- 1½ lb. Yukon Gold potatoes, unpeeled, cut into ½" pieces
- 1 bunch beets, trimmed but not peeled, scrubbed, cut into ½" pieces
- 1 medium red onion, cut into ½" pieces
- 1 large turnip, peeled, cut into ½" pieces
- 1 head garlic, cloves separated, peeled

Preheat oven to 425°F. Lightly coat 2 large rimmed baking sheets. Combine all ingredients in a large bowl. Divide vegetables between prepared baking sheets; spread evenly. Sprinkle generously with salt and pepper. Roast vegetables until tender and golden brown, stirring occasionally, about 1 hour 15 minutes.

SUGAR SNAP PEAS

123 calories

Serves 4—123 calories per serving

- 2 cups sugar snap peas, washed
- 3 T. olive oil

Heat the oil in a skilled over medium heat. Add the peas; cover and steam 3 minutes. Remove lid and stir, allowing peas to lightly brown, about 2 minutes.

CRISPY POTATOES WITH WILTED ARUGULA

90 calories

Serves 4—90 calories per serving

- 1½ lb. small Yellow Finn or red-skinned potatoes
- 8 large cloves garlic, cut into ½" dice
- 2 T. water
- salt and freshly ground black pepper
- 1 cup finely chopped young arugula
- ¼ medium onion, minced
- ⅓ cup white wine vinegar

Start potatoes in cold water to cover. Simmer until tender enough to be pierced with a knife but not falling apart. Drain and cool. Slice the potatoes about ½" thick. Lightly film the bottom of a 12" sauté pan with olive oil or cooking spray. Add the garlic and water and warm over medium-high heat, then turn the heat to low, cover, and cook 20 minutes or until garlic is soft but not browned. Remove the garlic with a slotted spoon and reserve.

Turn the heat to high and, standing back so as not to get spattered, add the potatoes, sprinkle with salt and pepper, and turn gently to coat with pan juices. Then spread out in a single layer and sauté until golden brown on the bottom. Turn and take to golden brown on the other side. Add the green and onion and cook over medium-high heat 1 to 2 minutes, turning frequently. The greens should wilt and begin to crisp. (Alternately, you could hold back ½ cup of the chopped greens, folding them into the finished dish off the heat.)

Quickly add the vinegar and scrape up the glaze at the bottom of the pan, taking no more than 30 seconds. Immediately turn out of the pan onto a serving plate. Sprinkle with the reserved garlic, taste of seasoning, and serve at room temperature.

SOUTHERN SUMMER SQUASH

111 calories

Serves 4—111 calories per serving

- 2 T. butter
- 1 large sweet onion, sliced into rings
- 8 yellow summer squash, sliced
- ½ tsp. salt
- ⅛ tsp. pepper

Melt the butter in a skillet. Add the other ingredients. Cook over medium heat until the squash cooks down and the onion begins to brown, stirring occasionally, about 30 minutes. When done, the squash is soft and takes on a golden color.

RED CABBAGE WITH CRANBERRIES

65
calories

Serves 10—65 calories per serving

- 1 small head red cabbage (about 8 cups)
- 1 T. olive oil
- 1 large onion, thinly sliced
- 1 cup dried cranberries
- 3 cups water
- 1/2 tsp. salt
- 1/4 cup red wine vinegar
- 1/4 cup agave nectar (or 1/3 cup Splenda or alternative granular sweetener)
- 1/2 cup orange juice
- 1/2 tsp. allspice
- 1/4 tsp. cloves

Core the cabbage; shred or chop and place in a bowl. Cover the cabbage with cold water. Set aside. In a large pot, heat the olive oil over medium heat. Add the onion and cook until translucent. Add the remaining ingredients. Bring to a boil and then reduce heat to low, simmering for 50 minutes to an hour. Stir occasionally. Cabbage will be tender and most of the water will be cooked out.

ARTICHOKE STUFFED TOMATOES

107
calories

Serves 6—107 calories per serving

- 6 large ripe tomatoes
- 1 (14 oz.) can artichoke hearts, drained and rinsed
- 2 oz. cream cheese
- 1/4 cup Parmesan cheese, grated

Preheat oven to 400°F. Cut tops from tomatoes. Carefully remove pulp with fingers, then remove core with sharp knife, being careful to leave the bottom of the tomato intact. Place in a greased baking dish. In a medium bowl, mash artichoke hearts with cream cheese and Parmesan cheese. Press gently into the tomato shells, mounding any excess mixture on top. Sprinkle each with Parmesan cheese. Bake for about 35 minutes or until tops are lightly browned. These may also be cooked on a covered, medium-hot grill, but place around edges rather than directly over flame. Serve on a lettuce-lined dish for a pretty presentation.

LOUISIANA RED BEANS & RICE

190 calories

Serves 8—190 calories per serving

- 2 (9.5 oz.) packages dried red kidney beans
- 1 large onion, coarsely chopped
- 1 stalk celery, chopped
- 2 garlic cloves, minced
- 4 scallions, chopped
- 2 bay leaves
- 1 tsp. dried thyme leaves
- 1 tsp. ground red pepper or more to taste
- 1 tsp. Worcestershire sauce
- 2 quarts cold water
- salt to taste
- 4 cups cooked long-grain white rice for serving
- ½ cup finely chopped fresh Italian parsley plus additional for garnish
- hot red pepper sauce as an accompaniment

Soak the red kidney beans overnight in cold water to cover by 2". Or quick-soak beans by bringing them and enough cold water to cover by 2" to a boil over moderately high heat in a large kettle; boil for 2 minutes, remove the pan from heat, cover, and let stand for 1 hour. Drain the beans in a colander.

Lightly film a Dutch oven with olive oil or cooking spray. Add the onion, celery, garlic, and scallions. Cook, stirring, for 10 minutes. Add the soaked beans, bay leaf, thyme, red pepper, Worcestershire sauce, and 2 quarts of water. Bring to a boil and simmer over very low heat for 3½ hours, adding a little more water if necessary, until the mixture is thick and the beans are very tender. Season to taste with salt. Remove the bay leaf. Mash some of the beans together until the entire mixture is creamy. For each serving, spoon 1 cup of beans over ½ cup rice. Sprinkle parsley on top and serve hot pepper sauce on the side.

CHERRY COMPOTE

- 1¼ lb. large bing cherries, stems removed
- ¾ cup Chardonnay
- 3 T. sugar
- ¼ cup cherry jam
- 1 tsp. cornstarch dissolved in 1 T. water
- 1 T. kirschwasser (a cherry flavored spirit, optional)
- 4 T. light sour cream
- cookies (optional)

Pit the cherries and reserve the pits. Place the pitted cherries, wine, sugar, and jam in a stainless-steel saucepan. Arrange the reserved cherry pits on a piece of plastic wrap set on a cutting board and cover them with another piece of plastic wrap. Using a meat pounder or the base of a small heavy saucepan, pound the pits to crack them. Place the cracked pits in a piece of cheesecloth and tie them into a compact package. Add this package to the cherry mixture in the saucepan. Bring the cherry mixture to a boil, cover, reduce the heat to low, and boil the mixture gently for 5 minutes. Add the dissolved cornstarch and mix well. Cool. Stir in the kirshwasser, if desired. Serve the compote in glass goblets with 1 T. of sour cream on top of each serving and, if desired, a few cookies.

BAKED PEACHES WITH BERRIES

- 4 ripe peaches
- fresh raspberries or blueberries
- 8 tsp. brown sugar
- 4 tsp. lemon juice
- 2 tsp. unsalted butter

Preheat oven to 350°F. Halve peaches and remove pits. Place peach halves in a baking dish just large enough to hold them. Fill the tops of the peaches with raspberries or blueberries or a combination of the two. Sprinkle the brown sugar and lemon juice on top. Dot with butter. Bake approximately 45 minutes or until the peaches are nicely browned and tender when pierced with the point of a knife. Serve warm or at room temperature.

BAKED PEACHES WITH ALMONDS

- 4 ripe, firm peaches (1½ lb.)
- 2 cups water
- ¼ cup maple syrup
- 1½ T. light brown sugar
- 1 T. unsalted butter, broken into pieces
- ⅓ cup whole unblanched almonds
- light sour cream (optional)

Preheat oven to 350°F. Using a sharp knife, cut the unpeeled peaches in half and remove the pits. Arrange the peaches cut side in one layer on a baking dish. Add the water, maple syrup, brown sugar, butter, and almonds. Place the baking dish on a cookie tray and bake for 40 minutes. Turn the peach halves so they are skin down and cook them another 15 minutes (at this point the juice around the peaches should be syrupy). Turn the peaches carefully in the syrup so they are skin up again and cool them to room temperature. Serve with the syrup and top with a dollop of light sour cream.

PLUM COBBLER

Dough Topping

- ⅓ cup old-fashioned rolled oats
- ⅓ cup all-purpose flour
- ⅓ cup sugar
- ⅓ cup pecan halves
- ½ tsp. ground cinnamon
- 3 T. unsalted butter
- 1 T. canola oil

- 1¼ lb. (about 7) ripe plums (Santa Rosa or Friar)
- ⅓ cup sliced dried apricots
- ½ cup plain yogurt or light sour cream

Preheat oven to 400°F. For the dough topping, place all the dough ingredients in a bowl of a food processor and process the mixture for 15 to 20 seconds, until it is crumbly. Quarter the plums and pit them. Place the plums in a 6"-cup baking dish and distribute the apricots around them. Sprinkle the dough mixture on top. Bake the cobbler for 40 minutes. Serve lukewarm with a tablespoon of yogurt or sour cream on top.

MANGO, LIME, AND COCONUT MOUSSE

- 1½ lb. mangoes
- 1½ tsp. unflavored gelatin
- 3½ T. fresh lime juice
- 2 T. sugar
- ¼ tsp. coconut extract
- ½ cup fat-free evaporated skimmed milk
- 2 T. flaked coconut
- fresh mint sprigs for garnish

Place a small bowl in the freezer to chill. Peel the mangoes and cut the flesh from the pits. In a small saucepan, sprinkle the gelatin over the lime juice and let stand for 5 minutes. Place over low heat and stir until the gelatin dissolves, about 1 minute. Remove from the heat. In a food processor or blender, combine the mangoes, gelatin mixture, sugar, and coconut extract and process until smooth. Pour the mango puree into a large bowl. Remove the chilled bowl from the freezer and pour the evaporated milk into it. Using a whisk, beat until thick and foamy, about 5 minutes. Fold the evaporated milk into the mango puree just until no white streaks remain. Divide the mousse among four ¾-cup bowls. Cover and refrigerate until set, about 6 hours. While the mousse is chilling, preheat the oven to 350°F. Spread the coconut in a small pan and toast in the oven until golden, about 3 minutes. Remove from heat and let cool. Just before serving, remove the mousse from the refrigerator and sprinkle each serving with the coconut. Garnish with mint.

NECTARINE AND PEACH GRATIN WITH CINNAMON SABAYON

- 3 large peaches, halved, pitted, and each cut into 12 wedges
- 3 large nectarines, halved, pitted, and each cut into 8 wedges
- 1 cup (4 oz.) blueberries
- ¾ cup sweet Muscat wine
- 3 T. honey
- 3 eggs
- 1 T. minced orange zest
- ¾ tsp. ground cinnamon

In a large bowl, toss together the peaches, nectarines, and blueberries. Divide the fruit evenly among six 1-cup gratin dishes and place on baking sheet. Preheat the broiler. Pour water to a depth of 3" into a saucepan and bring to a simmer over medium heat. Meanwhile, in a heatproof bowl, whisk together the wine, honey, eggs, orange zest, and cinnamon. Place the bowl over (not touching) the barely simmering water in the pan. (Be sure to cook the egg mixture over simmering, not boiling, water. Otherwise you end up with custard instead of a light and frothy sabayon.) Whisk constantly until the egg mixture triples in volume and is thick and foamy, about 8 minutes. Remove from the heat and spoon over the fruit to cover completely. Broil about 4" from the heat source until golden, about 3 minutes. Remove from the broiler and serve at once.

Note: Any combination of ripe fruit, particularly juicy summer fruit, may be substituted.

CINNAMON WALNUT COOKIES

Makes 5 dozen cookies—76 calories per cookie

- 2 cups walnuts
- 1 cup whole grain pastry flour
- 1/2 cup low-fat or defatted soy flour
- 1/2 cup oat bran
- 1 tsp. ground cinnamon
- 1/4 tsp. salt
- 1 cup butter, softened
- 2/3 cup fructose or Whey Low D granules or 3/4 cup Splenda

Preheat the oven to 300°F. Place the walnuts, flours, bran, cinnamon, and salt in a food processor using the sharp blade. Briefly process the mixture, just until the nuts are finely chopped and evenly mixed. Set aside.

In a medium bowl, cream the softened butter. Add the sweetener and beat until fluffy. Beat in the egg until thoroughly mixed. Add the dry ingredients to the butter mixture and stir until evenly mixed.

If desired, line your baking sheets with parchment paper. Otherwise, use ungreased baking sheets. Taking walnut-sized pieces of the batter, roll the cookie mixture into 1"-diameter balls and place each on the baking sheet, placing them about 2" apart. Using a fork, gently press each cookie to about 1/4" thickness. Drag the tines of the fork across, leaving lines in each cookie.

Bake 15 minutes. The cookies will be lightly browned. Cool a few minutes, then gently slide a spatula beneath each to loosen. Move to a rack or flat surface to finish cooling. If you used the parchment, slide the whole thing onto your countertop after loosening.

FIG BARS

173 calories

Makes 16 (2") bars—173 calories per bar

Filling

- 2 (8 oz.) packages dried figs
- 2 cups water
- 1/4 cup fructose or agave syrup
- 1/2 tsp. cinnamon

Crust

- 1 cup whole wheat flour
- 1/2 cup unsweetened coconut, grated
- 1/2 cup oat bran
- 1/2 tsp. salt
- 1/2 tsp. baking soda
- 1/4 cup Splenda or granular alternative sweetener
- 1 tsp. cinnamon
- 6 T. butter, softened
- 1 egg, beaten with 2 T. water

In a medium saucepan, place all the filling ingredients and simmer over low heat. Cook about 3 hours, until the figs are tender and the consistency of paste. Add water during cooking as needed. Cool. Process in a food processor or blender. The filling may be made up to two weeks ahead. Store in a refrigerator until ready to use.

To make the crust, combine the dry ingredients. Add the softened butter with a pastry blender or fork. The dough should be crumbly. Pour the egg mixture into the center of the dough and mix with a fork until the dough holds together. Divide the dough into two halves. Spray an 8" square pan with nonstick spray. Press half the dough evenly into the bottom of the pan. Spread the fig mixture evenly. Crumble the remaining dough over the top, then pat together so the figs are covered. Bake at 350°F for 30 to 35 minutes, until the top is lightly browned. Slice into squares while hot, then cool before removing from the pan.

Unleash Your Greatness

AT BRONZE BOW PUBLISHING WE ARE COMMITTED to helping you achieve your ultimate potential in functional athletic strength, fitness, natural muscular development, and all-around superb health and youthfulness.

Our books, videos, newsletters, Web sites, and training seminars will bring you the very latest in scientifically validated information that has been carefully extracted and compiled from leading scientific, medical, health, nutritional, and fitness journals worldwide.

Our goal is to empower you! To arm you with the best possible knowledge in all facets of strength and personal development so that you can make the right choices that are appropriate for *you.*

Now, as always, **the difference between greatness and mediocrity** begins with a choice. It is said that knowledge is power. But that statement is a half truth. Knowledge is power only when it has been tested, proven, and applied to your life. At that point knowledge becomes wisdom, and in wisdom there truly is *power.* The power to help you choose wisely.

So join us as we bring you the finest in health-building information and natural strength-training strategies to help you reach your ultimate potential.

FOR INFORMATION ON ALL OUR EXCITING NEW SPORTS AND FITNESS PRODUCTS, CONTACT:

Strength & Honor

BRONZE BOW PUBLISHING
2600 East 26th Street
Minneapolis, MN 55406

BRONZE BOW PUB

WEB SITE
www.bronzebowpublishing.com

612.724.8200   Toll Free **866.724.8200**   FAX **612.724.8995**

ANYTIME. ANYWHERE. TOTAL STRENGTH & FITNESS FOR MEN & WOMEN.

Imagine a complete strength and fitness program that slims, shapes, and sculpts your entire body in just 20 minutes a day. A program you can do anytime and virtually anywhere. A program so complete it requires no gym and no exercise equipment. Best of all, a program that covers every muscle group from your neck to your toes and delivers visible results in as little as 3 weeks.

Using the revolutionary Transformetrics™ Training System that utilizes time-tested body sculpting techniques along with high-tension Isometrics that literally allow you to become your own gym, *The Miracle Seven* offers:

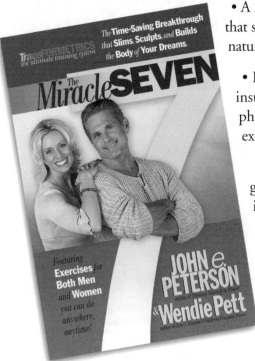

• A 20-minute per day weekly plan that sculpts the entire body to its own natural perfection.

• Detailed day-by-day exercise instruction, fully illustrated with photos that show each and every exercise.

• A special "speed it up" program that accelerates fat-burning results for those who want to see their results yesterday.

• A comprehensive nutrition plan that allows you to lose body fat faster than you gained it while providing easy to follow guidelines for eating healthy.

• The exhilaration that comes from knowing that you have complete control over your body, your life, and your destiny!

CREATE THE BODY OF YOUR DREAMS, transform your health to vibrancy, and extend your youthfulness without the requirement of a gym or expensive exercise equipment or fad diets, and do it anytime and anyplace.

Trans**FORMETRICS**
the ultimate training system

No matter what your present size or shape, *Every Woman's Guide to Personal Power* will guide you step by step through the most effective exercise system ever taught. Whether your goal is to drop a few pounds, shed several dress sizes, or to sculpt the body of your dreams, you will find everything you need to help your body achieve its natural, God-given strength and fitness potential. And it can be done in the privacy of your own home!

If you've never exercised in your life, or if you're an athlete looking to maximize your daily work-out, here are the exact strategies and methods you need. Precisely illustrated with 100s of detailed photos showing every facet of every exercise, you'll never have to guess if you're doing it right. Feel what it's like to have twice as much energy as you've had in years and in less time than it requires to drive to the gym and change into exercise clothes.

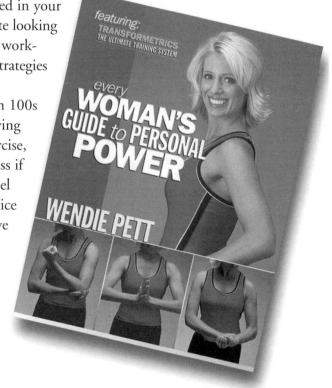

IF YOU'VE BEEN LOOKING FOR AN EXERCISE SYSTEM that will give you the results you've always dreamed of having, does not require either a gym or expensive exercise equipment, can be done anytime and anyplace without requiring an outrageous commitment of time, you're holding it in your hands.

Based solidly upon the most effective exercise systems as taught by Earle E. Liederman and Charles Atlas during the 1920s, *Pushing Yourself to Power* provides you with everything you need to know to help your body achieve its natural, God-given strength and fitness potential. Whether your desire is simply to slim down and shape up, or to build your maximum all-around functional strength, athletic fitness, and *natural* muscularity, you will find complete training strategies specifically tailored to the achievement of your personal goals.

The **Ultimate** Do It Now
Do It Anywhere
Lambs to Lions
Complete Guide to Total Body
Transformation

PUSHING YOURSELF to POWER

JOHN e. PETERSON

Precisely illustrated with 100s of clear, detailed photos showing every facet of every exercise, you'll never have to guess if you're doing it right again. You'll achieve the stamina you've always wanted in less time than it requires to drive to a gym and change into exercise clothes. Feel what it's like to have twice as much energy as you ever thought you'd have!

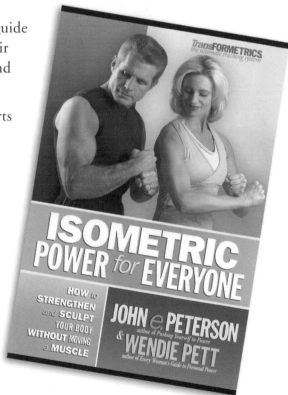

AWESOME STRENGTH AND A GREAT PHYSIQUE WITHOUT MOVING A MUSCLE

Isometrics, when done correctly, can reshape a person's physique and add strength beyond imagination without the person ever moving a muscle. By powerfully contracting the muscle in an isolation hold, a person can literally sculpt their body, shed fat, and rebuild nerve endings without ever having to go to a gym or lift weights. But the power of isometrics lies in being taught how to do them correctly.

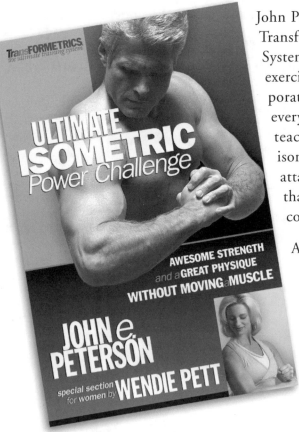

John Peterson, the creator of Transformetrics™ Training System, details the isometric exercises and how he incorporates them into his everyday life. Wendie Pett teaches how certain isometric holds are used to attack those trouble zones that women are especially concerned about.

Available fall 2005.